Offbeat Otolaryngology

What They Didn't Teach You in Medical School

John DC Bennett
BSc MB ChB BA MA FRCS DCH DHMSA

John Riddington Young
OStJ TD and bar MB ChB MPhil FRCS DLO

Thieme
Stuttgart · New York

Georg Thieme Verlag,
Rüdigerstrasse 14,
D-70469 Stuttgart, Germany
Thieme New York, 333 Seventh Avenue,
New York, NY 10001, USA

Printed in Germany by Gulde Druck, Tübingen

ISBN 3-13-128951-1 (GTV)
ISBN 1-58890-053-3 (TNY)   1 2 3 4 5

THE AUTHORS

John D C Bennett is an intensely shy and private individual who spends much of his time wondering why he has ended up where and what he is. In the past few years he has taken to travelling the world researching obscure medical curiosities and unsung heroes, with whom he is beginning to feel a strange affinity. His mother is very worried.

John Riddington Young is a ferret breeder, wood carver, arable farmer and Punch & Judy man who grows prize-winning sweet peas. His main hobbies are kite-flying, cricket-umpiring, otolaryngology and the Territorial Army. Like John Bennett, he is a Yorkshire Chauvinist but is at present doing missionary work in North Devon where he lives with a bull terrier, five children and his wife, who has always been very worried.

PERSONAL MESSAGE

Next to a personal knowledge of men, a knowledge of the literature of the profession of different countries will do much to counteract intolerance and Chauvinism. The great works in the department of medicine in which man is interested, are not so many that he cannot know their contents, though they may be in three or four languages. There is abroad among us a proper spirit of eclecticism, a willingness to take the good where-ever found, that augurs well for the future. It helps a man immensely to be a bit of a hero-worshipper, and the stories of the lives of the masters of medicine do much to stimulate our ambitions and rouse our sympathies.

I commend this book most heartily and wish the young authors every success.

Personal message from Sir William Osler (1849-1919) received in a dream by one of the authors (JDCB).

DEDICATION

The authors respectfully dedicate this slim volume to:

1. HM Queen Elizabeth the Queen Mother

    who is not only a constant source of inspiration but also Colonel in Chief of the Royal Army Medical Corps, in which both authors are proud to serve.

2. All poor and distressed bar maids, wherever they may be.

3. Alicia (Berlin, Stoke on Trent and Paris*).

    * a city in France

PROLEGOMENON

It is not necessary to know Latin, but merely to give the strong impression that one has forgotten it.

We perhaps ought to start by pointing out for the benefit of our American readers and those poor souls without the benefit of a proper classical education that *prolegomenon* is derived from the Greek *prolegein* (to say beforehand), and is a term used in scholarly books to describe prefatory remarks.

One of the reasons Dr Samuel Johnson gives for writing his dictionary is so that people will know how to spell *waistcoat*, the pronunciation of which had already become *weskit*, as shown in the Cockney rhyming slang "Jim Prescott" (perhaps American and Australian readers should skip this altogether and proceed directly to the next chapter). Our reason for writing this is to help junior colleagues to bluff their way in erudite otolaryngological circles and be able to give the impression that their ENT education has been properly rounded off.

Knowledge of fascinating trivia about a subject always gives the impression that the holder of this useless information is also privy to all the other important facts which are just too mundane to utter. At the apex of the petrous temporal bone is an almost imperceptible piece of fibrous tissue connecting it to the sphenoid bone. Below this so-called *petro-clinoid* ligament in *Dorello's Canal* (a channel formed by dura mater) runs the abducent nerve. Its immediate lateral relation is the *Gasserian Ganglion* which lies in another invagination of dura mater, *Meckel's Cave*. What a cornucopia of claptrap! Especially if you know who these worthy anatomists were - but it gets better: although apical petrositis from chronic suppurative otitis media must be about as common as rocking horse manure[a], it can be nonetheless confidently diagnosed if *Gradenigo's*

---

[a] In F.W. Watkin-Thomas' standard textbook of 1953 (London: H K Lewis) it was quoted as being "rare", with E.D.D. Davis seeing six in thirty years, the author recalling five in the same period i.e. the 1920s to the 1950s.

4

Syndrome is present! This is otitis media associated with diplopia from weakness of the ipsilateral external rectus muscle (caused by involvement of the abducent nerve in Dorello's canal), and ipsilateral retro-orbital pain due to irritation of the Gasserian ganglion.[2]

Is this knowledge useless? Not a bit of it. As Francis Bacon so succinctly put it: *"Nam et ipsa scientia potestas est"* - or *"for knowledge itself is power"*, and be advised that notwithstanding its rarity, Gradenigo's syndrome has already been asked no less than eight times in the Diploma of Laryngology and Otology and Fellowship of the Royal College of Surgeons exams. And that is just the written exams. Think of the one-upmanship when asked *"Just who is this Gradenigo, young man?"* and be able to be ready with the answer: Guiseppe Gradenigo from Naples was clearly not dearly enamoured by his colleagues. His obituary is a masterly Machiavellian tribute on how to damn your recently demised senior colleague with faint praise. Casually dropping this gem, implying of course that you have personally read the obituary should rattle up your viva score considerably.

One of the authors was asked in a Fellowship viva if he knew who Trotter (of Trotter's Triad) was; it should be pointed out that the patient under discussion did not actually have the three factors which Trotter had described and it was necessary to inveigle into the answer that Trotter's Triad was <u>not</u> in fact present! Not that failure would have been inevitable had it not been known, but once it was mentioned that *"Wilfred"* was from Gower Street, and then the dropping about his friendship with King George whose rib he had resected to drain a royal empyema when the official King's Surgeon had failed miserably to cure him - and, of course, his later refusal to receive a knighthood (in fact, he refused several times, preferring to be plain old *Mr* Trotter, which must be very confusing for our American and Australian readers - they should now immediately turn to page 115), the kindly pair of old gentlemen on the far side of the green baize table smiled benignly and all seemed plain sailing afterwards. Indeed, true interrogation ceased and the three chatted on about his amity with the King and how he would *"pop in for tea at the Palace"* through a special door in Buckingham Palace Road known only to members of the Royal Household and family friends. Then the bell went. This would not have been possible without our dear old chief, Kenneth Harrison, interrupting the dissection of a particularly pungent temporal bone one afternoon with the rather dramatic news that Trotter was a giant. That was all he said initially, *"He was a giant you know"!* It seemed that something nasty might have been going on

5

within his sella turcica[b], but then it was related that Trotter had been described as *"an artist with a knife"* and subsequently the vignette about the King's empyema was unfolded. It was the 12th Century monk, Bernard of Chartres, quoted on the title page of Shambaugh's *Surgery of the Ear* [3], who spoke of giants:

> *We are all like dwarfs seated on giants' shoulders If we can see a long way, it is not because we are tall, but it is because we are seated on giants' shoulders.*

The specialty of Otorhinolaryngology is not only well endowed with "giants" but has also provided the founders of two other specialties, paediatric surgery and plastic surgery. The former was developed by Denis Browne, known to all otolarynogologists for his development of tonsillectomy instruments, the latter by Sir Harold Gillies.[4]

That is not to say that things have always been rosy. Sir Astley Paston Cooper (1768-1841) had a deep interest in conditions of the ear and was awarded the Copley medal after reporting twenty of his cases to the Royal Society, but he soon retired from this work *"as he was afraid to be thought an aurist"*.[5]

Our distinguished predecessors have not confined themselves solely to the academic aspects of our specialty. George Cathcart (1861-1951) was always very interested in problems of the voice and suggested that in order to prevent vocal strain orchestral instruments should be tuned to French pitch and not to the higher concert pitch as was customary. In 1894 he founded and financed the first Promenade Concerts at the Queen's Hall, London, insisting that his friend Henry Wood should be the conductor.[6]

In summary, there are a lot of interesting things to learn about. Read on!

---

[b]

Sella Turcica or Turkish saddle. You may have spent many troubled hours wondering what a turkish saddle is. There are two main types of horse saddle nowadays: the English and the Western. The English saddle (formerly called Hungarian) is for more expert horsemen; the Western or "cowboy" saddle is, not surprisingly, bigger and has a pommel on the front to which one can tie one's lariat at rodeos. It used to be called a Moorish or Turkish saddle, the pommel being fancifully represented in the skull by the posterior clinoid processes. There are four clinoid processes because a *clinos* was a bed and of course had four posts (we also get the word *clinic* from this).

THE DEVELOPMENT OF THE SPECIALTY AND RISE OF HOSPITALS

In which the authors explore :

(a) The Ascendency of Specialisation

(b) Climbing the Ladder of the Specialty

(c) The Foundation of ENT Hospitals

(d) The Interface with Radiology

(e) The Role of the Fairer Sex

(f) The Role of the Church

(g) Fear and the Medical Profession

(a) The Ascendency of Specialisation

During the first half of the nineteenth-century most physicians were generalists who tended to look down on specialists as they were associated with quacks and itinerant healers who performed a single medical procedure. How very different things are today! Specialisation began to develop in the second half of the century on the ideological basis of the anatomic concept that disease attacked and resided in specific places within the body. This was coupled with the absolute increase in medical knowledge fuelled by the great advances made in pathology. Evil humours of vague provenance were replaced by a much more precise localisation of the seat of the trouble afflicting a patient. This process was stimulated by the multiplication of scientific instruments. It was the discovery and, more importantly, the publicising of the means by which indirect laryngoscopy could be performed that gave laryngology such a boost. Manuel Garcia's story is well recorded in standard texts, but what is perhaps not so well known is that articles on him on his 100th birthday appeared in both *The Strand Magazine*[7] and *Punch*[8]. The skilful use of such instruments required special education and practise, thus fostering specialisation. In addition to these medical and technological factors, the industrialisation and increasing concentration of the population into cities provided areas which could support specialised doctors.

It must, however, be remembered, that there were no barriers preventing such "specialists" from competing with generalists for patients, and many so-called surgeons were little more than general practitioners. The day books of Sir William Fergusson, who was to become Professor of Surgery, King's College Hospital in 1839 and Surgeon Extraordinary to the Queen in 1855 reveal that though busy with consultations and making over eighty visits to patients a month, he performed only two or three operations over the same period[9].This seemed to do him little long term harm, the *Lancet* writing: *"Few men equalled and probably none surpassed him as an operator"*.[10] The generalists faced not only competition from the specialists but also from hospitals and dispensaries which provided free care. To add to their troubles there were groups such as the practitioners of Christian Science, herbalists, and sellers of patent remedies, many of whom encouraged patients to treat themselves. As the reputation of specialists grew, patients would often visit them directly instead of relying on generalists to decide whether a consultation was necessary. Much of this might instil a distinct feeling of déja-vu to the British reader of the 1990s who is beginning to hear similar questions being raised. As these pressures continued there came about an economic disparity between generalist and specialist practice and also between that found in rural areas with practice in the cities.

At the International Medical Congress of Brussels in 1875, eight sections represented the state of scientific medicine at the time; for the Paris Congress of 1900 there had to be seventeen.[11] In 1910 the surgeon William Mayo warned that interdependence was an inevitable consequence of medical growth owing to the fact that the sum total of medical knowledge was now so great. In the United States of America an attempt at an alternative to the unifying knowledge provided by a brilliant clinician was found with the proposal to link specialists through formally organised co-operative medical associations. This co-operative specialisation reflected the tendency toward group effort that characterised industry and various social enterprises in the early twentieth century. Although by the 1920s such co-operative approaches to medical care were integral to the functioning of the hospital, it was actually doing more to foster specialism. Other branches of Medicine have not been immune to change and expansion. In 1900 there were no more than 305 Fellows of the Royal College of Physicians of London. By 1940 there were 619, and in 1992, 5,736. Members of the College, primarily trainees, rose from 452 in 1900 to 17,616 during the same period. This is especially important when one bears in mind that at the beginning of the century there were only two royal colleges in England - that of the Physicians (founded 1518) and the Royal College of Surgeons, which although with a history dating much longer, only received a royal charter in the nineteenth century. Only one further college emerged before the Second World War, the Royal College of Obstetricians and Gynaecologists which began in 1929. The two other colleges had attempted to prevent this, fearing they would lose their monopoly on qualifying exams, an important source of revenue. In 1952 the Royal College of General Practitioners became established, despite further opposition from the Physicians, to be followed by the Royal College of Pathologists. This was particularly important for this specialty, which feared *"becoming mere drudges, purveyors of reports"*.[12] Of course there are now colleges of radiologists, psychiatrists, anaesthetists and ophthalmologists. One wonders whether there will ever be one for otolaryngologists and in this we are reminded of the dream experienced by His Holiness the Pope, John Paul II. He spoke to God, posing the question as to whether the Church would ever be reunited. The reply came that it would, *"but not in your lifetime"*. He then asked whether women would ever be ordained into the Roman Catholic Church. God replied again that this would come to pass in the future, *"but not in your lifetime"*. For the final question of the three he had been allowed he asked whether there would ever be another Polish

Pope.   The deity replied:
        Not in my lifetime.

How, in fact, do specialists come about? Put simply, they possess either skills, such as special techniques of treatment, or have access to special equipment denied the generalist. Of course there is an overlap - the surgeon is unlikely to be able to exercise his surgical prowess without the requisite facilities - which were more and more being provided solely within the hospital setting. Specialties such as radiology developed purely by the expediency of controlling technical equipment, though even with this seemingly straightforward case we find that in the early years many generalists who had enough money to buy the kit lost no time in setting themselves up as "specialists".

Otologists had been appointed within British hospitals by 1851 but were primarily physicians, as were laryngologists. In 1872 William Dalby (1840-1919), who in 1900 founded the Otological Society of the United Kingdom, was appointed the first aural surgeon to St George's Hospital, London.[13] In that same year, 1872, that doyen-to-be of otolaryngology, Sir Henry Trentham Butlin (1843-1912) was surgical registrar to St Bartholomew's when the "registrarship" was a relatively new appointment.[14] In fact the Committee of Westminster Hospital announced in 1870 that registrars *who have hitherto done the duties of these appointments gratuitously will be remunerated; the sum of eighty pounds has accordingly been voted for the purpose, but only for the ensuing year.*[15] The British Rhino-Laryngological Society was formed in 1888. Sir Felix Semon[c] (1849-1921) was the first laryngologist to be appointed to a general hospital, in 1882, to St Thomas' Hospital (in London)[16] and established "subsection" status for laryngology at the International Medical Congress in London 1881. Full status was obtained at the next meeting in Copenhagen.[17] However the *British Medical Journal* of 1905 records how plans were laid to boycott the International Medical Congress to be held in Lisbon in 1906 as *"the Organizing Committee have placed laryngology, otology and rhinology as one subdivision".*[18] To add insult to injury, dentistry formed the other part. Attention was drawn to the fact that on 13th January 1905 the Laryngological Society of London had reaffirmed the resolution passed in 1902 that at all international medical congresses laryngology and otology should both be assigned a full and separate section. It was decided that in default of a definite assurance that laryngology should have the position

---

[c] Born in Danzig (now Gdansk), he served in the Prussian Uhlan guards and saw active service during the Franco-Prussian War 1870-71.

to which it is entitled, the delegates would take no part in the Congress. The dentists' view on all this is not recorded but readers should perhaps remember that for a long period throughout post Second World War Great Britain there was only a handful of professors of otolaryngology. It is somewhat ambiguously claimed that F C Ormerod in 1949 "was appointed the first professor of Laryngology and Otology in the first Chair to be created for our specialty in this country".[19] Professor Victor Lambert never had an established chair in Manchester. Phil Stell hat a title a while before a full-time academic post was set up at Liverpool. Nevertheless this is considerably less than the Chairs in dentistry in any one dental school.

At the beginning of the twentieth century the problems facing the specialty were addressed by Patrick Watson-Williams (1860-1938)[d]. Some of his thoughts might well be applied to the current debates over the training of members of our specialty towards the end of the century. Whilst recognizing that too early a specialization was to be avoided and that a sound up-bringing in the whole range of general medicine and surgery was the only safe foundation for any special branch, he resented the fact that there was a tendency to make another specialty (general surgery) the academic test of fitness. It is quite remarkable that in 1910 he was saying in his presidential address to the laryngological section of the Royal Society of Medicine that *"medicine was becoming a secondary consideration with a consequent danger of our becoming too exclusively surgical"*[20].

Sixty years later, the pioneer of hip replacement surgery, John Charnley, bemoaned the fact that the Royal Colleges could not find a formula to reconcile *"their obsession with a broad background of general training with the need to produce adequate numbers of highly competent surgeons"*.[21] He drew attention to the fact that existing qualifications were being denigrated, a fact only too well known to today's graduate who is suffering from the "academic inflation" which requires more and more post-nominal letters. As Charnley points out, every decade fewer and fewer postgraduates are regarded as completely trained to do the work required. In an attempt to prevent so wide a field of knowledge being required that it would be spread too thinly, what Charnley referred to as *"the British characteristic to prefer amateurism to the intense approach which leads to professionalism"*, he advocated more specialisation. Of course one must

---

[d] Who, incidentally, styled himself *doctor* rather than *mister*.

not forget that no matter which aspect of disease one studies one remains a doctor, and to the patient suffering from something which is to him unique and important it is essential that the humanity, courtesy and common sense which are so often squashed out of individuals during their training are not forgotten. This was brought to the author's attention by an article by a doctor describing the last days of his grandfather, admitted to a hospital for terminal care.[22] The grandson drew the houseman's attention to the fact that persistent vomiting had been treated only with oral antiemetics and there had been no control of his pain. The reply to this was that he was *"entitled to feel angry and distressed, and that analgesia would be discussed with the MacMillan team"*. The senior registrar later explained that *"they had wanted to give him every chance to recover before starting terminal care"*. Clearly we do sometimes get it wrong. Charnley deplored the situation where every surgical specialist had to pass the same postgraduate examination; in this, of course, he was concerned with orthopaedics. However the specialist otolaryngology FRCS exam was established only relatively recently (1947) and even so general surgery constituted a half. The situation in Britain is now changing but progress has been very slow. At present there seems to be no likelihood of our specialty receiving the status of a faculty within the various colleges of surgeons, let alone a separate college and in this respect the dominance achieved by general surgeons this century is likely to continue.

(b) Climbing the Ladder of the Specialty

Lionel Colledge (1883-1948) qualified in 1910 and the following year, at the age of twenty-eight was a fellow of the Royal College of Surgeons. Before the age of thirty he had been appointed assistant aural surgeon to St George's Hospital and assistant surgeon to the Hospital of Diseases of the Throat, Golden Square.[23] Even this rapid acceleration through the ranks can be bettered by William Daggett[e] (1900-1980)[f] who was appointed

---

[e]

Our American readers should take careful note not to confuse with the character *Little Bill Daggett* played by Gene Hackman in the film *Unforgiven* (Dir: Clint Eastwood, 1992. U.S. 131 mins Cat 15). Within British examination circles this might well consitute a *lethal error*.

[f]

Daggett had an idiosyncratic idea about mastoidectomy, believing the *anterior* epitympanum to be the most often neglected area of clearance during mastoid surgery.He described *Daggett's Angle* anterior to the head of the malleus and always paid great attention to exteriorizing this part of the cavity.

to the consultant staff at King's College Hospital, London at the age of twenty-eight.[24] This is just as well since that great medical man, Sir William Osler held that *"all progress was made, or at least started, before forty and a man should retire from active work at sixty"*. This was certainly the case for George Huntington, who described the disease known by his name in 1872, as the age of 21. He had become familiar with the genetic disorder during rounds with his father, a general practitioner on Long Island and this was his only contribution to medical research - like his father he was content in a country practice.[25] The authors would not like to imply that this constituted *"retiring from active work"* - but we digress.

It was noted in 1910 at the Presidential Address of the Laryngological Section of the Royal Society of Medicine that there was a tendency in Britain to:
carry on examinations unduly, and thus to trench too far on the precious years of early adult life, when a man's best original ideas are germinating and should be cherished and allowed spontaneous growth, instead of being trammelled and choked out of life by scientific pedagogy.[26]

What a strange idea!
    When proposals were carried in the *Lancet* in 1958 regarding cardiologists with one being appointed to *"every major hospital centre"* it was boldly declared that *"recommendations are made for a period of at least five years training after registration"*.[27] This rings with a rather hollow tone to those currently fighting their way from short-term contracts as "juniors" in the National Health Service to tenured posts many years after this period of time. Incidently, the same article ends with the rhetorical question that if specialties continue to "encroach", *"Has the hospital service of the future any place at all in fact for the general physician?"*. This was in 1958.

    Advice, often given with the best of intentions, can also mislead. The great surgeon Sir William Arbuthnot Lane, Bart had, whilst a student, set his heart upon the study of medicine and was not interested in surgery. He was appointed to Guy's hospital as a house physician and was befriended by one of the consultant staff, Dr Moxon, who pointed out to him that the prospects of progressing on the medical side were remote; that he, Fagge, Wilks and Pavy were strong healthy people, likely to live a long time.

However he considered that every member of the surgical staff at this time suffered from some condition likely to shorten his life. Consequently Lane devoted himself to the study of surgery, determined to overcome his repugnance of it. How wrong Moxon's forecast was is shown by the fact that owing to the deaths of Fagge, Wilks, Moxon and Pavy, Dr Hale White, who was a year younger than Lane, was appointed to the medical staff in 1886, two years earlier than Lane was appointed assistant surgeon![28] Of course, when it comes to climbing the rungs of any professional ladder, more is required than the convenient death of one's superiors and rivals. There is that indefinable quality which in some allows a characteristic to be used to advantage, whilst others are damned by it. The diligent reader will find many examples of this in the ensuing pages.

(c) The Foundation of ENT Hospitals

From the last third of the eighteenth century there was a new development - the foundation of medical institutions by medical men. These special hospitals played a key role in confirming the position and power of specialists.[29] In the words of an 1860 edition of the *British Medical Journal* they enabled medical men to *"step to fame and fortune by means of bricks and mortar"*.[30] The fact that they could be a route to power, prestige and wealth is underlined by the vociferous opposition they encountered from much of the medical profession in the mid-nineteenth century. Despite this initial condemnation, by the end of the century, those aspiring to the top of their specialty were applying to join the staff. To set this in some sort of historical context one must remember that in the eighteenth and nineteenth centuries the middle and upper classes were usually treated at home, with hospitals generally being supposed only for the *"deserving poor"*. Senior doctors would give of their time free of charge in exchange for the prestige and contacts which accrued from such an association; junior medical men used hospitals in order to learn their craft.

Initially these were usually simply outpatient departments, based on that started by John Lettsom in 1770. He was also the founder of the Medical Society of London, from which the Royal Society of Medicine developed. What might be considered the first British hospital specialising in otology was set up in 1816 as a dispensary in Soho Square by John Harrison Curtis (1778-1860) who began his professional life as a dispenser in the Royal Navy. From these humble origins as the *Dispensary for Diseases of the Ear* arose the Royal Ear Hospital which is now part of University College Hospital, a humble teaching hospital in London.[31] The specialist hospitals evolved from these outpatient dispensaries and, once in, the doctor had access not only to wealthy governors and patrons but the basis on which to establish a practice. As an indication of the value of such a position it should be noted that at John Lettsoms's Aldergate Dispensary two competing applicants paid six hundred guineas between them to secure an entrance.[32] The template for otolaryngology was Moorfield's Hospital, founded in 1805 by John Cunningham Saunders (1773-1810).[33] It was originally for both the eye and ear, but treatment of ear conditions ceased after two years.[34] Saunders was born in Devon and, after being apprenticed to a barber surgeon, walked the wards in London and became house-pupil to Sir Astley Paston Cooper. Following this, he became a lecturer at St Thomas' Hospital, no doubt paying for the privilege. However, when his mentor left for Guy's Hospital in 1800, taking on Benjamin Travers as his apprentice, Saunders was left out in the cold. He departed for the provinces the following year. He was in luck, however, for having worked for Astley Cooper, he could draw on this connection by emphasising a degree of specialisation in otology by publishing a book.[35] In 1804 he established his *London Dispensary for the Relief of the Poor Afflicted with Ear and Eye Diseases*. This was clearly the thing to do - a check of the Medical Directories of the period reveals that by the 1860s there were at least sixty six specialist institutions in London alone.

The loyalty extended to a hospital might reach almost ridiculous proportions. A patient was seen at the Manchester Ear Hospital complaining of a running ear, which was treated. When an attempt was made to examine her other ear, this was refused. This ear was under the care of another hospital, St John's Dispensary just around the corner! The effort of attending for daily dressings at two different hospitals can be imagined and for those who cannot picture the chaos of the waiting room of such hospitals then Lowry's *Outpatients at Ancoat's Hospital* is an apt visual description. This picture used to hang in the hospital in Ancoats and was coveted by a well-known lady Minister of Health in the 1960s for her Whitehall office. For those of our readers who knew Manchester in the past but have not been back for some time, we have to relate that many of these neighbourhood areas have now changed quite a lot. This has not necessarily been for the better, not obviously for the worse - it all depends on one's needs. The corner tobacconist is now in the hands of a chocolatier. This is an advantage for those requiring something more than a bar of *Fry's Five Boys Chocolate*; it would prove difficult to get five Woodbines though. The new shop is clearly more profitable - "Art Deco" chocolate is

15

sold at a vast sum per ounce - it is simply *Toblerone* with the wrapping taken off. The shop next door is for futons. This is fine if your idea of living is to eat/wear/drink/(or whatever one does) to a futon[g]. The bolder of your authors enquired at a bespoke corsetry shop but remained unenlightened; at least we know it is nothing to do with that. Perhaps for once our American readers can turn the tables and enlighten us?

Of course the concentration of cases in such specialist hospitals led to a wealth of clinical experience for the otologists working there. Sometimes the unwitting testimony of the local inhabitants showed the extent of ear disease within the community. This was demonstrated to one of the authors when a Salford woman brought one of her many children complaining that *"his left ear won't run properly"*. That ear was the only one in the whole extended family which had an intact tympanic membrane. Whilst demonstrating a new instrument he had devised for tonsillectomy Mr J F O'Malley told the audience that he was in the habit of operating on thirty cases in the morning at his hospital in two hours.[36] Whilst the cases may have been concentrated together in specialist hospitals, the specialists may well have found themselves covering a very wide area indeed. George Archer was appointed in1932 to be consultant to Manchester Northern Hospital and Stockport, Buxton and Warrington Infirmaries.[37] Similarly,Lennox Browne (1841-1902) seemed to work in London, being aural surgeon to the Royal Society of Musicians and surgeon to the Royal Choral Society; he was in addition to this also consultant to Newcastle Throat and Ear Hospital.[38] E D D Davis was appointed to the senior surgical staff of Charing Cross Hospital, London but was also on the staff of the Royal Dental Hospital, the Throat Hospital, Golden Square, the Hospital for Sick Children, Great Ormond Street, Mount Vernon Hospital and Queen Alexandra Military Hospital, Millbank. In between commuting he managed to find time to do some operating and also to be President of both Sections of Laryngology and Otology of the Royal Society of Medicine.[39]

The rationalisation of a multitude of small hospitals into fewer "more efficient" units is nothing new. Prior to the outbreak of war in 1939 the Central London Throat, Nose and Ear Hospital amalgamated with Golden Square Hospital to become the Royal National Throat, Nose and Ear Hospital. Chapple Gill-Carey (1896-1981), who had

---

been appointed to the consultant staff of the Central in 1923 became the first Dean of Laryngology and Otology, a post which he held until 1960. Robert Scott Stevenson (1889-1967), a former Manchester registrar, ex Royal Army Medical Corps and writer, saved the independence of the Metropolitan ENT Hospital at the post-war inauguration of the NHS.[40]

(d) The Interface with Radiology

The close liaison which has developed between radiotherapy and ENT is, of course, a reflection of the fact that squamous cell carcinoma is the commonest nasty in the upper aero-digestive tract and on the whole is eminently radio-sensitive. Wally Jackson, a radiotherapist from Norwich tells the story of Professor Ralston Patterson, the first director of the Christie Hospital and Holt Radium Institute, Manchester on a ward round where one of his firmly held views was challenged. Ralston did not give much truck to the time-honoured idea that clay pipe smoking gave rise to cancer of the lip. (One of your authors who used to smoke a clay pipe as a schoolboy vividly remembers tearing the skin from his own lip after it had stuck like glue to the white stem of the pipe. A new pipe always had a red lacquer over the mouth piece but this became easily broken off). The director, firmly convinced of the error of this theory, was somewhat put out to learn, on enquiring of the smoking habits of a patient with a fungating lip cancer, that he did in fact smoke a pipe, and, even better, a clay pipe. However, not to be put out, Ralston asked him on which side he smoked it. The patient, who had a large tumour on the right side, looked puzzled but pointed to the left side.

"What did I tell you?"

announced the Professor, triumphantly.

"Here is a man who has smoked a clay pipe all his life on the right side of his mouth, and then goes and gets cancer of his lip on the other side!"

A discussion ensued as to how best transform the appearance of the man's mouth to something resembling a kebab (or hedgehog) by the intelligent use of radium needles and then, before moving on, the Professor asked if any of the students would like to pose a question of their own. One lad, a little less overawed by the situation than many, asked the old Lancastrian[h]

"Have you always smoked your clay pipe on the left sir?"

The reply came:

"Oh no! I always used to smoke it on the right until this bloody thing came along".

A *dewlap* is the hanging pouch of flesh found at the throat of oxen and dogs. It is present because the investing layer of cervical fascia in their necks is not attached to the Adam's apple (so called because a piece of the forbidden fruit of the tree of knowledge of good and evil became stuck in his throat causing this swelling; this theory has been challenged recently) as it is in humans. A *radiation dewlap* is a sequel to late-stage tumours of the tongue, pharynx and supraglottis, well-known to ENT surgeons and radiotherapists alike. Nevertheless it had been described neither in standard texts nor journals until a bright spark seconded from ENT to radiotherapy collected a few cases. He found that if the dewlap was pressed with the thumb for a few minutes it behaved like pitting oedema. It was duly written up and one of your authors now has two academic prizes for describing in print what everybody already knew. We call it Riddington Young's sign.[41]

Neville Samuel Finzi (1882-1968) was a pioneer of radiation therapy and director of the X-ray department at St Bartholomew's Hospital. He worked with Harmer on the application of radium to the larynx via needles inserted through fenestra in the thyroid cartilage.[42]

(e) The Role of the Fairer Sex

Florence Cavanagh (née Nightingale) died at the age of eighty-four, having been a consultant at the Royal Manchester Children's Hospital. She graduated MB BS in Melbourne in 1933 [43] and was a firm believer in the importance of washing out the

---

[h]

From the county of Lancashire, one of the foremost English counties and the provider of three kings in succession during the Wars of the Roses. It is surpassed only slightly by its more illustrious neighbour, Yorkshire.

sinuses of all children who suffered from glue ear - a legacy which is still followed by many who drank from the fountain of ENT knowledge in Manchester. Long after her retirement, when one of her disciples was questioned on the practice of performing antral lavage on every Mancunian child listed for myringotomies the answer given to your author was:

A sinus lavage is less invasive that irradiating a child's head, young man!

Unabashed, the enquirer then had the temerity to point out that it was only seldom that he had found any abnormal washings. To this the reply came that he wasn't looking properly and that he should hold the glass syringe up to the light to see the yellow crystals glinting back! After that if the sinus lavage proved clear the operation note was annotated *crystals*.

Esme Hadfield was an undoubted "giant". Some purists may well take issue with this, saying that we should call her a giantess, but those who knew the late great Esme will know full well that she would have preferred giant. Witness the fact that she always got changed in the "Surgeons' Changing Room" at High Wycombe Hospital, pointing out that she considered it quite inappropriate for her to use the "Nurses" as she was a surgeon and not a nurse. She was the co-opted member for many years on the council of the BAOL but eventually gave it up because it was a *"rights balls-ache"!* Apart from that, of course, "giantess" gives the strong impression that there may be something lurking within the sella turcica. Esme, who died only recently, was a highly respected member of the profession and established, by her own footslogging and door-to-door visiting of remaining relatives, the causal relationship between adenocarcinoma of the nose and hardwood dust in the local furniture industry in High Wycombe.

Of course women have not always had it easy. It was reported in 1893 that the Faculty of the Colombian University in Washington decided to close its doors against female medical students for the reason that *"the presence of women kept students of the sterner sex away"*. Furthermore the authorities had *"no desire to transform it into a female seminary"*.[44] In 1902, the Senate of the University of Göttingen unanimously decided not to allow women students to matriculate.[45] Certainly the courtesy and welcome with which they are invited to join the profession have not always been as effusive as is currently found. Indeed an editorial in the *Journal of the American Medical Association* as recently as 1886 remarked that:

One effect of this higher education of women, of which we hear and read so much, will be to hinder those who should be good mothers on men from being mothers at all... A good professional education is very expensive;...not alone of money, but of physiological force. Every woman cannot be a mother, wife....But it is not assuming too much to say that woman was born to marry and bear children....There are some women who must work, and if they cannot find woman's work to do then they must work as best they can, even as men. But there is now a tendency to turn a woman into a man as a sort of experiment or fad.....Parents, teachers, and the family doctor should endeavour to repress this growing tendency. If our girls were taught the true physiology of woman this tendency would be in a great measure stopped.[46]

This was written when a Russian princess living near Kiev was ten years old. It is a good thing she never read it otherwise Princess Dr Vera Gedroits might never have qualified in medicine, served not only in the Russo-Japanese War and First World War but also as personal medical attendant to the Russian Imperial Family and ended up in 1929 as Professor of Surgery.[47]

To avoid getting bogged down in the tedious arguments about whether the fairer sex is adequately represented by numbers in the otolaryngological world the authors would like to point out that there are more ENT surgeons in Greater Munich than in the whole of the United Kingdom. This expresses far more eloquently than their humble efforts could convey their position which remains, as it has always been, to support right, fight wrong and defend the weak.

(f) The Role of the Church

In the entrance of the Royal National Throat, Nose and Ear Hospital in Gray's Inn Road the more observant visitor may have noticed a rather nice idol to St Blaise, the patron saint of diseases of the throat. Aetius of Amida, on the Tigris (ca AD 500-550) gives not only one of the best descriptions of ENT diseases to be found in ancient literature but the first reference to St Blaise. His full recommendation was to:

Bid the patient attend to you and say "Bone (or whatever it is) come forth, like as Christ brought Lazarus from the tomb and Jonah from the whale". Then take him by the throat and say "Blasius, martyr and servant of Christ, saith, 'Either come up or go down.[p]

20

He was also called Blasius or Blazey and there is not only a town in Cornwall named after him but also a church next to the toy museum in Salzburg. Your authors were first made aware of him since he is also the patron saint of woolcombers and there are pubs in Yorkshire and other wool producing areas called *The Bishop Blaise* [i]. Prior to becoming the Bishop of Sebaste in Cappadocia (now Armenia) he was a physician and had also evidently found time to invent the woolcomb. During a purge on Christians by the Emperor Licinius in 289 AD he was imprisoned, and whilst in gaol miraculously cured a boy with diphtheria from fatally choking. This, however, did not impress his captors overmuch who decided to tear the flesh from his limbs with an iron woolcomb and then, just to be on the safe side, to behead him.[48] The statue in Gray's Inn Road shows him before this happened. Finian Houlihan informs us that in Ireland children to this day take red scarves to be blessed on St Blaise's Day with the hope of avoiding illnesses of the throat. In like manner, one of your authors as a young man always used to make a silent devotion to Venus, goddess of love, when ever placed in a situation when he needed, but did not have, a condom [j].

A legend frequently illustrated by mediaeval artists is the impregnation of the Virgin Mary through the breath of the Holy Ghost in her ear (showing that perforations of the ear drum were well known from earliest times). Following on from this we could consider an ear defender to be an early form of contraception.

The speech defect of Moses is widely interpreted as stammering. It has received a full and scholarly appraisal by S Levin[49], and there is little further that your authors can add save to remark that as he never took part in any broadcasts where time was at a premium (remember that even now the Levantine is not usually noted for his adherence to tight schedules) it would not be as great a handicap as for someone such as Billy

---

[i] The reader is cautioned to avoid stumbling into the trap of thinking that the word *blazer* is in any way related; to do so would be to commit what the authors are led to believe is known in examination circles as a "lethal error".

[j] This was replaced for a while by the Triple Alliance method of contraception which consisted of the triad of frequent hot baths, tight underpants and always giving a false name and address.

Graham [k] in modern times. Levin does not touch on this at all.

One of the roles of the Church has always been considered as a repository for knowledge; the literary abilities of monks and other clerics has long been held in high esteem. Sometimes, unfortunately, mistakes are made and scientific and literary gems come to light after languishing for centuries, mis-indexed in the back rooms of the Papal libraries. The librarians, it must be remembered, were not "blessed" with modern technology such as computers. The Chair of Anatomy at Rome was held in the sixteenth century by Bartholomeus Eustachius (1520-74). His work was not published during his lifetime, otherwise it might have rivalled that of Vesalius, who was his conteporary in Padua. In particular, his account of the anatomy of the larynx is much more detailed and accurate - alas, it remained unnoticed until the eighteenth century when the copper plates of the illustrations were discovered in the Vatican library. The Roman nobleman Aulus Cornelius Celsus who lived in the first century AD wrote a medical encyclopaedia in eight books, *De Medicina* but this was lost until 1478 when it came to light once again in the Papal libraries. It was one of the first medical books to be printed, but of course poor old Celsus received no royalties.

The Venerable Bede reported in 685 AD that St John of Beverley restored the speech of a deaf and dumb man and was later made patron saint of the deaf and dumb.

(g) Fear and the Medical Profession

Fear takes many forms. What might appear terrifying to one individual may merely be the stimulus to another to achieve something worthwhile. However for those to whom a perceived threat is very real, actual fear is the opposite to that state of complete health so beloved of the World Health Organisation as including a feeling of well-being. As such, it can erode away the efficiency of the person and even his will to carry on. For the medical profession, fear has taken many forms, which over the years have changed as the challenges we face alter. An easy example is the fear of contracting the disease the patient we are treating is suffering from - a very real threat in times gone by. The very real risks of personal injury to which doctors in armed forces and attached to expeditions

---

[k]

Who of course was never challenged with any form of formal speech defect.

and the like cause fear of a very special quality. There is also the fear of personal failure, inadequacy and the tendency to feel responsible for the diseases and deaths of those whom we treat. Although not claiming to be exhaustive, the following examples, some of which are well known, review some of the fears to which members of the medical profession may be liable. Perhaps they will serve, if not as a guide, then as milestones with which to compare and contrast one's own experiences. Very little that one might experience has not happened to someone else before.

Moral Issues and the Courage to Fail

The fear of being thwarted in one's progress by stepping out of line and the challenge to question what one considers to be wrong is something which we expect in totalitarian regimes. History is full of doctors with strange-sounding names who have been exiled or sent for psychiatric treatment for this. One of the most famous names in English medicine may well have had his career blighted for this very reason, though fortunately his place in history has been secured. However, even now, apologists hold that *"there was in Hodgkin's nature that which made it hard for him to obtain ultimate success in life, some perverse spirit that seemed always to place him in opposition"*.[50] We prefer to think that he fell foul of the hospital "general manager", the one who held the purse strings and hired the staff. Let us review the obituaries in the *Lancet* of Hodgkin and Babington. They appeared on the same page, some thirty years after the appointment of physician at Guy's Hospital for which they had been rivals:

> *He had naturally looked forward to succeeding to the office of Physician; to his great mortification however, his claims were passed over, and Dr Babington, whose death occurred within a few days of his own, obtained the post, at that time almost entirely in the gift of the treasurer of the hospital.*

The penultimate paragraph of Babington's obituary reads:

> *It may appear to many, and, perhaps not unreasonably that the extent of Dr Babington's practice as a physician, as well as his general reputation, hardly come up to the above summary of his works and acquirements ;......if he was not brilliant, he was most kind to his patients.*[51]

Damning praise indeed! The *British Medical Journal* was even more forthright in its condemnation of Babington:

> *He was elected assistant-physician; overcoming on that occasion his opponent*

Dr Hodgkin, to whom long and assiduous labour had given strong grounds for competing for the honourable post....in 1840 he became full physician, with Drs Richard Bright and Thomas Addison - men whose names are historical in medicine - as his colleagues. He does not appear to have lectured much.[52]

What was the reason for Hodgkin's career being prematurely terminated, for he resigned all his hospital posts the day after the election? Hodgkin had an interest in the native Indians of North America and asked his colleague Dr Richard King, who was undertaking an expedition there, to find out as much as he could. His report was far from complimentary, and may be considered a nineteenth century indictment of multinational companies and their involvement in the Third World [1]. Hodgkin campaigned on the Indians' behalf against the Hudson Bay Company. Unfortunately for him, and he knew this at the time, the Treasurer of Guy's was a deputy governor of the Company. He was also a governor of Guy's.....

There are, happily, examples where those with the courage of their convictions have been rewarded. In fact the development of cardiac surgery and many advances in other specialties only occurred because someone had the courage to fail. The heart had been a forbidden organ following the great Billroth's pronouncement that a surgeon who tried to suture a heart wound deserved to lose the esteem of his colleagues. There is no beating about the bush here and it must have been with some trepidation that the young surgeon Ludwig Rehn sutured a stab wound in the right ventricle - and succeeded.[53] One can only conjecture how the German surgical establishment might have viewed a possible defence he could have used had he failed, the words of Peter the Great:

> *when in their youth they had trembled before the rod of their superiors and been praised only for servility?*

Mortal Danger

Fear of physical injury is not an emotion one might expect to be common within the profession in that, unlike the profession of arms in which one's calling is the infliction of violence, the situation, usually, within medicine, doesn't arise. However, life can be unpredictable. The call of the bugle in wartime can stir otherwise quite passive doctors

---

[1] Our American readers would probably consider the United States to be now part of the *First World.*

into a military role, or they can be conscripted. The peace-time military medical services may provide a means of obtaining professional qualifications or advancement not otherwise attainable.[54] At least it provides secure employment, but not all those serving expect to see action and those who leave after their time is up, and are then called back for some emergency, are presumably equally taken off their guard. Actuaries have little role to play in the assessment of risks to life or limb in war, important though they may be in the life assurance business. Diseases have traditionally caused far more deaths and casualties than weapons, but it is bullets and shrapnel which cause the fear and medals are given for plucking the few from the jaws of death rather than the many by preventive medicine. During the First World War in the battle of the Somme, doctors went out with their stretcher bearers in close support of their men across no-man's land. The cost was high - forty-three infantry battalion medical officers were killed.[55] Within days of chlorine gas being dispersed across the trenches in 1915, rudimentary gas masks were produced which by the end of the war had reached a high degree of sophistication. Yet lime packers in the North West of England alkali industry had stoically withstood this peril since mid-Victorian times. It took a war to alert the nation, and then within a very few days gas masks were being produced. It pays to have a high profile. A casualty officer attacked in a District General Hospital will probably not achieve the same headlines as his colleague injured on an oil rig, in the same way that rail crash injuries are far more newsworthy than those involving cars. One hopes that equal attention is paid to aiding the victims and preventing their recurrence, though this didn't happen to the poor old lime packers. It is a sobering thought to realise that for a medal to be awarded the act of bravery must be witnessed and an appropriate citation written. Acts of heroism without an audience are unlikely to be very rewarding. The Royal Army Medical Corps has more than its fair share of Victoria Crosses, but surely the supreme example of conquest of fear must be those two military doctors who, having won the Victoria Cross, went on to achieve a second. A less militaristic example, yet involving military doctors is the research into the transmission of yellow fever. There are many cases of experimentation, often with the researchers being the subject but this case of 1900 is important in that it was the first thoroughly controlled clinical research and it established the highest standards of informed consent.[56] Walter Reed had deep concern over the whole affair and described carefully the risks, from which one of the original four man team died. This weighed heavily on him for the rest of his life (he died in 1902) and when, in January 1901, his work was coming to its triumphant conclusion he wrote to the Surgeon General:

> *The responsibility for the life of a human weighs upon me very heavily just at present and I am dreadfully melancholic.*[57]

25

The Fear of Failing to Achieve Fame

Much is spoken these days about the pressure to publish if one is to achieve any progress within the medical profession. It might be a surprise to some that this is no new phenomenon, and many famous names in medicine suffered identical pressures in their formative years. This is a theme we will develop further in the chapter *Education And Training*. The requirement for a curriculum vitae to bear an impressive list of publication is nothing new. The fear of a gap in the requisite box or page is probably for many an equal inducement to publish as the love of disseminating knowledge. How galling when one passes an idea to a colleague, or worse, a friend, who subsequently makes use of it. This happened to Sigmund Freud, who as the reader will find when he reaches the end of this book, was made aware at an early stage in his career the value of a lot of publications. This does not, it must be noticed, always hold true. Korotkoff wrote in 1905 but a single paragraph describing his system for measurement of systolic and diastolic blood pressure - the sum total of his publications on the subject.[58] He found success, despite the opinion of the *British Medical Journal* of that year that by sphygmomanometry *we pauperize our senses and weaken clinical acuity*,[59] and we still remember the sounds as sounds of Korotkoff. As a young hospital doctor, Freud was forever short of money, so much so that he had to have a prolonged engagement as he simply could not afford to get married. To hasten this he sought means by which he could advance his career and thereby acquire private practice. It is somewhat ironic therefore that an opportunity for visiting his fiancée, from whom he had been parted for some time, caused him to stop his experimental research. This was on cocaine. His own account of the events of 1884 read:

> *I hastily wound up my investigation of cocaine and contented myself in my book on the subject with prophesying that further use for it would soon be found. I suggested, however, to my friend Königstein, the ophthalmologist, that he should investigate the question of how far the anaesthetising properties of cocaine were applicable in diseases of the eye. When I returned from my holiday I found that not he, but another of my friends, Carl Koller (now in New York), to whom I had also spoken about cocaine, had made the decisive experiments upon animals' eyes and had demonstrated them at the Ophthalmological Congress at Heidelberg. Koller is therefore rightly regarded as the discoverer of local anaesthesia by cocaine, which has become so important in minor surgery; but I bore my fiancée no grudge for her interruption of my work.*[60]

However, all was not immediately smooth for Koller following Freud's unwitting gift to him. He had limited himself to the eye, recruiting friends to pursue other application as he wanted to "establish a claim to the much coveted position of an assistant at one of the large eye clinics". Not unnaturally he was convinced that through this important contribution he was almost guaranteed a post in Vienna. But it was not to be. The following year he was involved in a fight with a colleague and had to leave his native Austria, losing his opportunity of obtaining the position of *Assistant* and his hopes of an academic career. It was during this period that Koller became depressed...[61] In 1888 Koller emigrated to New York, where he won many distinctions, including being several times proposed for the Nobel Prize. But Freud achieved fame of his own.

THE GENTLE ART OF BOUGINAGE AND ENDOSCOPY

In which the authors explore :

(a) The Development of Means by which Hitherto Secret Parts of the Body Came to be Revealed.
(b) The TRUTH about Linda Lovelace's Relations, Revealed for the FIRST Time through a Thorough Investigation of the FACTS.

(a) The Development of Means by which Hitherto Secret Parts of the Body Came to be Revealed.

It used to be said of the ENT Surgeon that he was the one chap who was able to paint and decorate his front hall and staircase through the letter box. This may have been eclipsed somewhat by the advent of *SMIGs* - the Society of Minimally Invasive General Surgeons. To follow the analogy they are able to manage the landing and bedrooms also. They are the "keyhole" coves beloved of the tabloid newspapers who are forever achieving breakthroughs, managing cholecystectomies through tiny holes and then sending the patient home on the bus at tea time, after admitting another one two days pre-op to block the bed and prevent it falling into the hands of the physicians or orthopaedic surgeons. This used to happen on the aural ward of the Manchester Royal Infirmary where your authors both had the privilege of working. It was just too easy for the casualty officer to send every case he admitted there rather than laboriously telephone around the hospital because there were always beds available. That was until the advent of the M.R.I. FMed1. This was a form the size of an A4 sheet of paper with detailed questions covering both sides. Before the aural ward would accept a lodger this form had to be filled out. It usually proved easier to telephone around the hospital. Sadly, your authors never really got the credit their military training had taught them in the devising of this bureaucratic portcullis.

Anyway we digress from the important subject of *SMIGs*. It should be noted that the word *smegma* is Greek for soap and not cheese *(n.b. The Young Woman from Leith)*. Digression, yet again! Let us turn now to 1938, when Baumes presented to the Medical Society of Lyon *"a mirror the size of a two franc piece"* for the examination of the choanae and larynx, which just goes to show how the French have to reduce everything to monetary terms.

But long before this, Philip Bozzini (in 1806) described the first instruments to *"see around corners in the cavities of the human body"*. Unfortunately his fiendishly clever (shades of Captain W E Johns here; Ed) endoscope was literally one candle-power. Goethe's dying words in 1836 were *"Mehr Licht!"* and he might well have been describing the contemporary state of endoscopic lights. Apart from natural sunlight, candles, paraffin lights and oil lamps had all been tried but with little success. Then one night when Dr Ziemssen was at the Music Hall, he developed a plan: Thomas Drummond had invented limelight for theatres in 1816[m]; his light consisted of a block of lime heated to incandescence by two jets of gas, burning hydrogen and oxygen. This provided a soft brilliant light capable of being directed and focused. Its intensity was of great value for spotlights but it was also used for the realistic simulation of moonlight and sunlight. It was the spotlighting effect that Dr Ziemssen was interested in; he devised an unobtrusive little device for endoscopy which was a sort of cross between a pressure cooker[n] and a linear accelerator. The great disadvantage of theatre limelights was that they required constant supervision by a dedicated operator who could keep adjusting the block of lime and redirect the two gas jets. If this was not attended to in Ziemssen's Endoskope, then the drum exploded. As this did not inspire confidence, it did not catch on.

The invention of the electric light in the latter half of the nineteenth century kindled new hope, but like the course of true love, it *"ne'er ran true"*. One initial problem was that the first electric lights had a platinum filament, and in order to get this to glow one needed a generator powered by a steam engine. This all but precluded its use for domiciliary visits (with the exception surely of showmen and those members of the population in possession of a steam engine? Ed.). Another problem was that so much heat was generated that the first cystoscopes (Nitze-Leiter, 1879) and the modified nasopharyngoscope (Zaufal, 1880) needed continuous water-cooling systems.

In 1880 Stoerk used a water filled glass sphere called a water lens or a *cobblers sphere* to focus the light. Apart from the over heating and the steam generator problems, an Italian hypochondriac killjoy named Voltolini was causing *"undue alarm and despondency"* - (an indictable offence during the Second World War[o]) that electric light was bad for the eyesight not only of the practitioner but also the patient. With a name

---

[m]

Hence the term *in the limelight* originally referring to the centre stage, brilliantly lit up by the limelights.

[n]

A device constructed from metal for the preparation of food, which is heated under pressure.

[o]

Your authors have been able to find no proof to support the rumour that this conflict was started by Vera Lynn's impressario in an attempt to boost what had been a flagging career.

like Voltolini one would have thought that he would have been in favour of electricity, though it has been, and continues to be, the source of much disquiet amongst people who one would have thought would have known better. A landlady of one of the authors was convinced that baldness would result from his sitting too long at his books under a strong electric light. He took the advice, and retains his hair (just). As a result of Voltolini's ravings, electric endoscopes were hardly used during the last twenty years of the nineteenth century. With the turn of the century, however, relief was at hand, not only for Mafeking[p], but for endoscopic lights. It came with the invention of a miniature light bulb which did not overheat.

It can be seen that the development of invasive forms of surgery with safety was dependent upon technological advances. It is perhaps not surprising to us to find that the inventive minds of our otolaryngological predecessors quickly adapted current inventions and made quite a few of their own. Watson-Williams proudly announced his *New Electric Light Gag for use in Operating on the Facial Regions &c* at the section of laryngology of the Royal Society of Medicine in 1912, claiming that by means of a small 3 volt metallic lamp carried on a stem fixed to a Doyen gag good illumination produced from outside the field of vision could be obtained.[62] Major E B Waggett (1867-1939) brought back oesophagoscopy and bronchoscopy instruments from Freiburg (1906) and was the first to use them in Britain.[63] His "day job" was ENT specialist at Charing Cross Hospital but for recreation he held a commission in the Territorial Army, commanding a section in the City of London Field Ambulance.[64]

Pop Hastings did oesophagoscopies under local anaesthesia and his patients would probably qualify afterwards as sword swallowers. They were sat on a three-legged stool and Pop Hastings, who had achieved fame as a fighter ace in the First World War (now sometimes abbreviated by those with a trivial outlook on life to WW1) and who also had a "day job" as a Member of Parliament, achieved his nickname of *Corkscrew Charlie* by encircling his seated patient as he advanced the oesophagoscope down the

---

p

A town in South Africa whose name has now, irritatingly, been changed to Mafikeng; (this has been added primarily for our American readers; clearly every true British otolaryngologist will be only too well aware of the lifting 17 May 1900 of the siege which began 12 Oct 1899). A quick straw poll amongst some of the younger (and, it must be admitted, female members of our specialty) showed that not everybody was aware, however, that the relief of Mafeking led to the coining of the term *maffick*.

gullet.

Practitioners who have as part of their professional duties the peering down of narrow pipes must always be wary of what might come at them in the opposite direction. This caution was not exercised by the officer who was inspecting the rifles of the men under his command for cleanliness. Those of our readers who have had military experience will know that this is performed from behind, with the rifle being held at the port position, the inspecting officer looking into the breech. On this occasion (a true story), the young subaltern peered down the barrel to see if it was clean. Still looking down the barrel he said *"Is it loaded?"* *"No sir,"* replied the man. *"Then pull the trigger,"* came the command. The private did so, and shot the second lieutenant dead.[65]

(b) The TRUTH about Linda Lovelace's Relations, Revealed for the FIRST Time through a Thorough Investigation of the FACTS.

No chapter concerning itself with the insertion of instruments into the aero-digestive tract would be complete without some mention of that heroine of the silver screen, Linda Lovelace. The authors, both of whom have qualifications in the field of historical research[q], do not understand, however, the widely held misconception that her grandmother went down on the *Titanic*; this is simply not supported by close scrutiny of the casualty lists.

---

[q]

As indeed did that larger-than-life character from the world of otolaryngology, Draffin. He refused to attend the final hearing of the General Medical Council into whether he should be struck off or not, claiming that he was far too busy reading Gibbon's *Decline and Fall of the Roman Empire*. He was struck off.

ANAESTHETIC CORRELATES

In which the authors explore :

(a) The Blossoming of the Art of Anaesthesia Under the Tutelage of Otolaryngology

(b) Why Anaesthetists Should Remember Draffin

(c) The Day the Balloon Went Up

(d) The Surgeons' Scissor-Jaw Reflex

(e) Madness and Anaesthesia
    and Much Much More

(a) The Blossoming of the Art of Anaesthesia Under the Tutelage of Otolaryngology.

It can also be the case that members of our specialty have learnt something from the anaesthetists. The authors cannot vouch for the autheticity of the following, but it certainly has the ring of truth about it. It concerns the case of the patient who attended the ENT Outpatient Department for a consultation and was advised that an operation would be necessary. She asked how long the waiting list was for such a procedure and was told that she would probably have to wait about a year.

> *How long then if I paid and went privately?*
> *When did you last have anything to eat or drink?*

(b) Why Anaesthetists Should Remember Draffin.

A full report of this appeared in the Christmas edition of the *Journal of Laryngology & Otology.*[66] It was also reprinted by *Today's Anaesthetist.* It would be "tearing the arse out of it" to reproduce it yet again in these pages.

Draffin is not the only member of our specialty to have had an interest in anaesthetics. Terence Cawthorne's fame as an otologist from Yorkshire tends to overshadow his ability in other directions. As well as being very interested in medical history (he was president not only of the section of the Royal Society of Medicine but also of the Historical Society of King's College Hospital) his earliest professional interest was in anaesthesia. He held the post of senior house-anaesthetist at King's College Hospital in 1929 and for many years following this he delighted in teaching the art of anaesthesia. It was said that throughout his life he retained not only a critical appreciation of anaesthesia but also sympathy for the anaesthetist in times of difficulty.[67] If this was indeed true then it makes a welcome change, for anaesthetic-surgical relations are not always happy and productive.[68]

(c) The Day the Balloon Went Up.

This is the story of a afternoon experienced by one of the authors which he would not care to repeat for a *very* long time. Being, as it is, worthy of the best adventure books, we reproduce it in full with the kind permission of the editor of *Today's Anaesthetist*, in which journal it was first revealed to the anaesthetic fraternity and the world.[69]

It *seemed* the normal sort of fraught day with which we are all familiar. Two surgeons and a couple of nurses all scrubbed up, not an anaesthetist to be seen but evidence of activity in the anaesthetic room. Little were we to know that we might well have become involved in a drama of explosive proportions, and with nobody to witness the final event, scattered as the potential witnesses were in the various walled-off areas (which were to assume such importance later on) from which modern operating suites are formed.

The over-stimulated memory cells are still a little fragile, but I think we were discussing some aspect of audit (in parts of our theatre we speak of little else), when I was amazed to notice that the balloon on the anaesthetic trolley was rapidly growing in size. Anybody who has watched television, and for practical purposes this means *everybody*, knows that the little black balloon is meant to inflate and deflate rhythmically with the patient's breathing. Hence the old anaesthetic cry *"Squeeze the bag!"*. When the black balloon stops, the alarms start beeping, the line on the monitor goes flat, and the credit titles and theme music start rolling. This is about the extent of the public's interest, but, as a surgeon, I know more. The balloon should not continue to grow. Especially as there was no patient hitched up to it. There was nothing connected to it except some lengths of tubing. Something was wrong. I pride myself on being a bit of an anaesthetist, chiefly through a thwarted love affair in the past which involved a lot of looking through those little glass porthole windows into the induction room. I don't claim to know very much - you know the sort of thing - all the little syringe, half the big syringe (but slowly). She really was so pretty I could have watched her for ages. But in essence, as an anaesthetist I am little more that a dabbler. I just know the basic FRCS stuff we surgeons have to learn to be safe. Like knowing that in the event of some catastrophe like the anaesthetist keeling over a staff accident form must be completed in triplicate. I can do that sort of thing with the best of them. But here we are talking of a disaster of massive proportions. Two surgeons and two nurses about to be either engulfed in rubber or blown to smithereens as the walls of the balloon gave way in an explosive decompression. An operative mortality of 400% - and no operation!

I have had a little military training so gathered the rest together and led them behind the solid wall which separated the scrub-up area from the operating area, sending out my

2IC[r]. My reasoning was that he might be able to shut off the supply of gases feeding the monster; failing that if he turned the wrong knobs, we might at least be able to spend our last few moments semi-anaesthetised. Disconnecting a few cables seemed to have no effect and we were all preparing ourselves for the inevitable (the scrub up area is a cul-de-sac and I had unwittingly been the leader of victims into what might have turned out literally into a dead end), when we were saved. There is a *shut off valve*. A technician, alarmed perhaps by the ominous quiet following the curtailment of our audit discussion, had come in. He deftly dealt with it in the correct manner, restoring the gases from the balloon to their correct receptacles.

There is no mention whatsoever on the anaesthetic machine (which appears not unlike the flight deck of Concorde) about this, nor is the current medical literature any help. I will make it my business in future to draw the attention of any new surgeon to this *valve*, and commend your readers to also adopt this habit.

(d) The Surgeons' Scissor Jaw Reflex.

A *British Medical Journal* article by one of the authors revealed this phenomenon to the world.[70] Once again, it would be "tearing the arse out" &c.

(e) Madness and Anaesthesia.

From Manchester, we can pass on the rather alarming tale of the mentally deranged sculptress who heard voices telling her that to atone for her sins she must strike out her eyes. Being as she was, armed with a chisel, it was the work of moments only for her to comply with this request. She was duly admitted to hospital spurting blood from two cavities beneath her forehead where her eyes had previously been. Before being taking to the operating theatre for some form of clean-up operation, the anaesthetist told her that it would be impossible for her sight to be restored but that the operation should control the bleeding; first it would be necéssary for him to anaesthetise her and that

---

[r] Second in command

38

would involve a tube being put down her throat. She ordered him to be very, very careful - for one of her front teeth had been capped!

(f) And Much Much More.

The great Killian had little requirement for the skills of the anaesthetist when he was performing his varied intubations, considering that:

> *an anaesthetic is only necessary in the case of children; local anaesthesia is preferable in adults, and is obtained by painting the pharynx, the aditus laryngis, the left sinus pyriformis, and especially the posterior cricoid region, with a 20 per cent solution of cocaine. For direct laryngoscopy excitable patients receive a hypodermic injection of morphia twenty minutes before the examination is begun.*

He goes on in his careful description of the requirements for direct examination without general anaesthetic to remind the reader that not only must the tube be oiled but also *warmed*.[71]

It has often occurred to the authors that it must be difficult for a visitor to an operating theatre to identify the different players in the surgical orchestra. We ourselves have a reasonable idea who our colleagues are and in which specialty they work. Subliminally we identify the urologist by his preferring to be shod in Wellington boots and wearing an apron; the orthopaedic surgeon is disarmingly frank about not being very bright, but is quick to point out that he can lift heavy weights; the neurosurgeons may be found celebrating when a patient can, post-operatively, move all limbs in a semi-coordinated fashion. We would like to add the observation that the anaesthetist is the one who carries his pen fastened around his neck with a string. Research has shown that these were the chaps who at school had their mittens securely tied together through the arms of their duffel coat. Our psychiatric advisers tell us that it is a form of insecurity and, like most things in life (according to them) dates back to early childhood and the fear of rejection by or loss of the mother. As doctors they fear losing the attention of the patient and are not really happy unless he is anaesthetised and will not run away.

LOTIONS, POTIONS AND PREPARATIONS

In which the authors explore, amongst many other things:

(a) The Role of Tobacco in Otolaryngology, Including a Prize-Winning Article

(b) Insights into Some Rare and Unusual Therapeutic Substances

(c) Some of the Early Writing into the Technique of Applying Substances Directly into the Circulation by Means of Venepuncture

(d) The TRUTH Behind Surgeons' Gloves

(a) The Role of Tobacco in Otolaryngology.

Tobacco has been used in the past both as a stimulant and a sedative, until it was found to have a toxic action. Enemas of tobacco smoke were administered through special bellows. It is quite remarkable to reflect how medical authorities have changed their tune regarding tobacco. But then again, considering that in the 1950s (the formative years for some very eminent professors and deans of today), the treatment for diverticular disease was a *low* fibre diet it is perhaps not so strange. There have always been people ready to legislate, though the *British Medical Journal*'s editorial of over a hundred years ago took the contrary stance from that taken today, namely:

> *There is a class of persons who employ themselves with all the energy of despair in raising some cry of alarm, and making everybody about them unnecessarily uncomfortable. They parade their bugaboo with a desperation which ensures a temporary public attention, and, as soon as this dies out, they start another of a still more attractive appearance.*[72]

Well that certainly applies to many pressure groups of today, but the criticism which follows is totally unlike the "holier than thou" food and health fads found in many current medical dictatorships:

> *The vegetarians would reduce mankind to live upon sky-blue and an apple, or at best an egg; the Maine Law liquor men would legislate all spirituous and malt liquors off the face of the earth; and now we are to have an anti-tobacco-smoking agitation, which is to end in the entire demolition of the "Stygian weed". It is quite clear that this restless class of individuals will not "let a body be", and we make thing ourselves lucky if hereafter we are not reduced by them to have our diet regulated by act of Parliament.*[s]

Let a body be, indeed. But when have doctors, and especially surgeons, been content to

---

[s] The reader will be pleased to learn that one of the authors received a cash prize for submitting this extract to *The Oldie* magazine for the section entitled *Voice From The Grave*. Views of his military medical colleagues varied from the opinion that only one as lazy as he would be so behind with his reading to be looking at an 1857 copy of the BMJ, to only someone so devoid of any consideration to the welfare of his patients would neglect them so and be reading &c.

do that? Tobacco has also been used as an adjuvant to mercury in the sweating baths for syphilis.[73] In fact there is a long history of treatment of venereal diseases with mercury, giving rise to the saying:

One evening with Venus, followed by a lifetime with Mercury.[74]

(b) Insights into Some Rare and Unusual Therapeutic Substances.

Mercury is not the only seemingly poisonous substance to be used in a therapeutic manner. Arsenic has also been used with profit and in fact Ehrlich's greatest practical success was achieved by the use of the arsenical compounds against trypanosomal infections. The anti-cancer drug *cisdiaminedichloroplatinum* is also a heavy metal *compound*.[75] In France, Lissauer used potassium arsenate in 1865 to treat chronic leukaemia. One would be mistaken if one were to think that practitioners in the past were totally unmindful of the potential for serious consequences of the therapeutic substances which they employed. Anyone adopting this line of thought has clearly not read the article which appeared in 1913 in *Semana Medica*, a deficiency which readers of this book can immediately rectify. For here one finds Botella writing about the effects of Salvarsan on the internal ear, or as he so charmingly puts it *Sobre los efectos del Salvarsan en el oido interno*.[76] He summarises eighty-one cases in which he examined the ears before and after Salvarsan treatment, recording nineteen cases of disturbances following its injection. His conclusion was that the drug should be given prudently, specialist examination of the ear should never be omitted, and all patients with a lesion of the auditory nerve should be excluded. The same care has not always be shown with potentially dangerous drugs, it must be admitted, and amongst these *ergot* must reign high. It was advocated as a treatment for epistaxis, swallowed as a liquid extract.[77] Other Victorian rhinologists preferred iron, plugging the nostrils with liquor ferri perchloridi.[78]

Acriflavine was used by C P Wilson of The Middlesex Hospital who put wedges soaked in the solution into the tonsillar fossae following a tonsillectomy. On being asked by NW Gill as to whether this was for haemostatic or antiseptic reasons he replied that it was so post-operatively he could tell by looking at the patients' lips whether he had performed a tonsillectomy or a sub-mucous resection. The technique is still continued in Manchester by D P C Canty (from whom both your authors received training), though not for this reason. Local acriflavine has been shown to be, in a concentration of 2 per cent, an effective and safe remedy for rhinoscleroma.[79]

There used to be a sister at the Manchester Ear Hospital, All Saints (known to Mancunians as the "Ear Hole") who would put in glycerine and ichthammol wicks for acute otitis externa. Instead of saying that insertion of the wick was no doubt a painful experience but the relief, once it was in place, was rapid, she would utter with an earthy northern laugh as she pushed the dressing in demure mill girls' ears:

It's like a lot of things in life this, pet; it hurts when it first goes in but once you've got it in you'll be pleased it's there!

Some Latin terms are not what they first may seem: *sordium coitus*, for example, could perhaps shock a man "with a little Latin". *Sordes* (from sordire, to get dirty) means, literally *"filth"*, and was used by our predecessors to describe *"the viscid matter discharged from ulcers, the black deposit on teeth etc"*. We assume everybody knows what *coitus* means (from co-ire, to come together[t]). Sordium coitus was the quite proper term for wax in the foramen of the ear [80] (the coming together of filth). The idea that cerumen (which is unimaginatively only Latin for wax) is filthy and not the wholesome bounty of a healthy ear canal packed with lysozymes and antiseptics, persists so that not only otologists but many generalists spend countless hundreds of man-hours per week trying to remove it. Foreigners are, needless to say, worse still, and it has not escaped the notice of one of your authors that each of the eight French _au pairs_ (other author's emphasis) to visit his home have left waxy cotton buds in his bathroom. He now considers that Johnson & Johnson Cotton Buds should have a health warning on the packet[u]. Further chaos can ensue when proprietary wax softeners are used in an attempt to loosen wax from the ear, especially when prescribed and dispensed by non-medical personnel. Your authors are aware of two cases where problems resulted from this. The first concerned a traumatic perforation following a water-skiing accident. The water masked the blood, and the perforation was not noticed because nobody looked.[81] The second involved a similar missed perforation but this time the powerful wax softener caused a facial palsy.[82] In India there are peripatetic wax wallahs who travel from door

---

[t]

Though, as we all know this might not always be the case!

[u]

During the late 1960s the rate of coronary heart disease in Finland was very high and thought to be associated with the high milk intake which was found there, most Finns drinking a pint or two of milk instead of beer with their evening meal. The Finnish government accordingly put a health warning on milk.

to door with a set of wax spoons, cleaning out the salubrious secretions for a few rupees. It is averred by our friend and colleague Suresh Shetty that they do a very good job. We hope that they don't confuse the spoons with those little ones which are used for the spices etc in the making of curry, though this is unlikely as this sort of job would be delegated to the memsahib. As an aside, we should perhaps mention here that in Oriental races, ear wax is grey rather than brown. Both your authors find it is unusual, but true, that Captain W E Johns in his long and detailed descriptions of the Simian appearance of many of Biggles' foes, never mentioned this detail.

The name *earwig* is interesting. The insect carries cerci, scorpion-like above its head when alarmed or aggressive; several species can fire a foul-smelling liquid formed in the abdominal glands for distances of up to ten centimetres. More interesting that this, though, is the name. It comes from the Anglo-Saxon *eare* and *wijca*. One hopes that the reader can guess the *eare* bit, but *wijca* is *"something which travels in"* (*vehicle* and even *way* share the same root). It was thought that this member of the Dermaptera order crept into the brain during sleep. *Forficula auricularis* have horny forcep-like tail filaments or *cerci*; these are pincer-like in the male, hence the origin of the French name *perce-oreille* (ear piercers), but not the Dutch which is *oorworm* or the German which is *der Ohrwurm*. However, this is used more often to mean a tune which one cannot get out of one's head. They also use *Ohrenkneipfer*, or ear nippers. The common thing to all these is that the word ear comes in. It is therefore no surprise that the Welsh for the insect is *chwilenglust* - clust being the word for ear (for the benefit of our American and Australian readers we should point out that it of course becomes glust when placed after an -en sound). In Hungarian, the verb *maszo* means to climb into; an earwig is a *fülbemaszo* and *fül*, would you credit it, is the word for ear. Over in the Near East, Turkish for earwig is *kulagakacan* and whatever a kulak was in Russia, in Turkey it means ear. Perhaps most amazing of all, and they do have earwigs in India, is that in Gujerati (𝒥𝑖𝜎 𝟧 ૬ 𝑖 𝗍 𝜀 𝒋) is earwig, and (𝑔𝑖𝜎) is ear!! Why, you may ask, is this association so widespread? It has been suggested that the pleated hind-wing when stretched out resembles a human ear! Your authors cannot somehow endorse this theory, which does not have the ring of truth to it. Can you imagine a primitive Turk (or Welshman) pulling the wings off an earwig? One of your authors wondered whether the tool used to pierce ears in the past looked like the sexual end of a male earwig. Incidentally, *Labia minora* is the name in the entomology book for the lesser earwig. *"found in nettle beds"* -your authors laboured under a completely different impression. A dictionary of European folklore avers that the insects *"crawl into your ears and eat your brains".*[83] The alleged cure is to lie down on newly turned-up soil, and the earwig will run out again. This could be a good way for medical practitioners to get their gardens dug.

Despite the fact that the humble earwig has this etymological association with the auditory canal neither of your authors has ever seen an earwig going into anything other than a Dahlia. They can end up elsewhere though - witness the unfortunate man who, after taking a sharp, deep, draught on his bronchodilator experienced a disagreeable and wriggly sensation in the centre of the chest. Following rapid and explosive coughing he managed to expel two earwigs.[84] Your authors must confess to a tremendous paucity of clinical experience when considering the earwig in the ear. Fortunately, our American cousins can relate two cases. The first concerns a postgraduate student in Flagstaff, Arizona who suffered a punctured and lacerated tympanic membrane.[85] The second concerns a patient who was much luckier - it was evidently a female which "cautiously emerged, to the relief of insect, child and father".[86] It cannot be said that such forays by the earwig are common. Not so with the cockroach (from the Spanish *Cucaracha*) which, according to *Encyclopedia Americana*[87] has a predilection for so doing. Between 1985 and 1989 the *New England Journal of Medicine* even contained, in an aptly named article, a "controlled trial" on *Removing Cockroaches from the Auditory Canal*[88] and a further piece comparing the use of lidocaine[v] and mineral oil[89]. What amazes your authors, who can remember tediously dissecting *Blatta orientalis* for their A-levels, is how the huge insects managed to get into ears in the first place, they are so big. Some attain a wing span of 5 inches. Another bug which definitely gets into ears and is evidently endemic in the ear canals of Navaho Indians, who sleep on untreated sheepskins, is the spinose Argasid sheep tick (*Otobius megnini*) which can cause severe perichondritis.[90] Of course the sheep themselves also sleep on untreated skins, but do not seem to be troubled by this problem. Why this should be so remains a mystery to your authors, who in the normal course of events are only too ready to embark on journeys far afield to sort out mysteries of an otolaryngological bent. In this case, however, neither felt any inkling to, in the words of our erstwhile colleague Andrew Salmon, live with shepherds and *find ourselves*. Probably because we do not consider ourselves as lost as him.

---

[v]

We think they mean lignocaine.

The casual reader (or American, Australian or whatever) who has not fully followed the authors' efforts to shed light and bring truth to some of the terms and descriptions used in otolaryngology may well be wondering whether such accuracy, bordering (as the uninitiated might consider) on the verge of pedantry, is really necessary. Of course it is! It is only through maintaining an ever-present vigil that Truth may shine through and the dark forces of Error and Sloppiness be banished. We applaud the courageous stand made by the editor of the *Lancet* who published the letter from the manufacturers of *Lysol* who were quite erroneously accused of being German. While not without serious consequences today, in 1914 such an unfounded accusation was totally reprehensible. For the benefit of our readers who may have been similarly misled and for that reason have not been able to fully enjoy the benefits of *Lysol*, we reproduce the letter in full:

> *Sir, - We are enclosing copy of several letters received from members of the medical profession who labour under the erroneous impression that we are a German firm trading in England. On the contrary, our principal is a loyal English-born subject, who has lived all his life in this country. Furthermore, all our staff are British, and there is no financial or moral relationship between our firm and Germany.*
>
> *Trusting that you may be disposed to publish these facts in the interests of fair play,*
>
> *We are, Sir, yours faithfully,*
>
> *For CHAS. ZIMMERMANN AND CO. (CHEMICALS), LTD*
>
> *O. A. Elias, FCS   Departmental Manager.*[91]

The use of substances therapeutic or otherwise is sometimes not without its dangers. Toynbee died at an early age whilst attempting to test the hypothesis that tinnitus might be relieved by the inhalation of the vapours of hydrocyanic acid and chloroform with a subsequent Valsalva inflation.[92] This was in 1866; had he lived until 1909 he might have died from snakebites after reading Politzer's description of the Annamite tribe in eastern India. They hold the belief that the ear is inhabited by a small animal and that tinnitus results from fights with similar animals - the treatment is fumigation with burning snakeskins.[93] The otological sophisticate should not be too disdainful of this, for

McNaughton Jones listed many pharmacological preparations in his textbook both as causes and cures for tinnitus.[94] Neither should the "moderns" amongst our readers be feeling too cocky, for in the Ciba symposium on tinnitus, Brown and his colleagues list drugs which may induce tinnitus, many of which are listed elsewhere in the same publication as offering relief from it.[95]

The packaging of modern-day drugs leaves much to be desired in comparison to their earlier counterparts, even if their therapeutic efficacy has been enhanced. This is not the only thing that counts, as anybody who has bought cosmetics or scent for a nurse can testify. The overall presentation is of supreme importance to the suggestible mind. That is why, of course, one of the authors gets away with sending *eleven* roses. The overall effect is just the same as a dozen and his parsimony is protected by two facts: first, what sort of girl would actually count? and second, she would simply believe that the shop had cheated him, thus making her all the more likely to forgive the transgressions which had necessitated their being sent in the first place. John Wilkinson is a retired haematologist who has a superb collection of Delft drug jars. The authors are evasive about his address, being no more specific than saying that he lives in the north of England, for the collection is worth a small fortune.

(c) Some of the Early Writing into the Technique of Applying Substances Directly into the Circulation by Means of Venepuncture.

The sleep-deprived resident tasked with prescribing and infusing a wide range of powerful antibiotics and cytotoxic drugs to wards full of head and neck oncology patients would find interesting the account written in the laryngological section of the Royal Society of Medicine during the 1910-11 academic year. It is entitled *Demonstration of Instruments for the Intravenous Injection of Salvarsan ("606")*.[96] One of the opening sentences will ring familiarly: "In making an injection into a vein, the great thing was to avoid putting any of the substance into the hypodermic tissue". However things did seem a little easier in those days in that:

> *The operator need not pay any attention to the tubes, leaving that to an assistant, his effort being to get the needle directly into the vein, after causing it to protrude by means of a bandage; taking care not to pass the needle through the vein*

beyond its farther side. The fact of being in the vein would be shown by the blood appearing in the glass.

(d) The TRUTH Behind the Surgeons' Gloves.

Whilst the preceding passage about the tribulations of achieving venous access in the past might, to the current surgical sophisticate, seem rather elementary, he should bear in mind the whole novelty of the procedure and the attendant anxiety which that can produce. The "operator" would have been able to wear rubber gloves, though it is doubtful whether he considered it necessary, HIV and hepatitis not being such a cause of worry as in current times. The history of the development of the rubber glove is interesting in that, unlike so much of what the authors have had to relate to the reader, this involves an episode of romance. Or at least this is the traditional story peddled to medical students about how Halsted, the first Professor of Surgery at Johns Hopkins Medical School in Baltimore noted that during the winter of 1889-90 the nurse in charge of his operating room developed a dermatitis from the solutions of mercuric chloride.[97] The Goodyear Rubber Company (which in the last decade of the nineteenth century was not too busy with car tyres and condoms) was asked as an experiment to make some thin rubber gloves for her. Sadly, the Goodyear Rubber Division of the United States Rubber Company has no record of them.[98] Of course the real story, which your authors will now divulge, is far more interesting than this rather soppy fairytale. On 10 January 1834 a young physician named Richard Cooke wrote a letter (now in the manuscript collection of the Rare Book Room of the New York Academy of Medicine, MS 560) in which he describes a *"very nice solution of Caioutchiouc, dissolved in Guthries spiritus of Terpentine"*. He described how after application the Terpentine evaporates......*"By lubricating the hands with it you have an insoluble pair of India rubber gloves - perfectly impenetrable to the most malignant virus"*.

This is the first known mention of rubber gloves *"in the surgeon's hand"* to prevent infection *"by the most malignant virus....in dissection rooms and in vaginal examinations"*. Just over a decade later an English physician suggested gloves for antisepsis.[99] Thus for a matter of several years before Ignaz Philipp Semmelweis had published his *Hochst wichtige Erfahrungen über die Aetiologie der in Gebaranstalten epidemischen Puerperalfieber* the English were being made aware of these immortal lines:

Whenever puerperal fever is rife, or when a practitioner has attended any one instance of it, he should use most diligent ablution; he should even wash his hands with some disinfecting fluid, a weak solution of chlorine for instance.....

The reader is exhorted, should he find himself in Vienna, to take himself along to the Institute for the History of Medicine there and relate this to the crone who is in charge of the department where Herr Semmelweis' washing bowl is kept like some Holy Grail. It drives her mad.

Cleanliness has not always been so straight forward and clear cut - in the past there a have been some ideas which sound quite strange to us now; who knows what dogmas which we hold so dear today will be ridiculed in the future? Powdered finely, tobacco was used as a disinfectant, and during the plague in England in 1665 the scholars of Eton were thrashed if they did not smoke before coming into the classrooms,[100] which brings us back to the initial theme of our chapter to which the reader is exhorted to return and reread.

AUDIOLOGY

In which the authors explore the world of audiology, including:

(a) The Early Development of the Subject

(b) The Scourge of Hearing Loss Caused Through Excessive Exposure to Noise

(c) The Development of Education of the Deaf

(d) Vertigo

(e) The Science of Audiometry

(f) The World of Hearing Aids

(a) The Early Development of the Subject.

In 5th century Greece, Alcmaeon and Empodocles (504-443 BC) knew absolutely nothing about the existence of the tympanic membrane but this did not in any way deter them from developing a theory of hearing. This was based on the idea that sound waves bounced round and round the convoluted cartilages of the pinna and then echoed down the external canal directly into the brain. Hippocrates, the so-called "Father of Medicine" (460-379 BC), knew full well, a century later, of the eardrum and modified the Empodoclean theory to include it.[101] He pointed out that only *"dry objects give off sound"*, hence the echoes from the dry tympanic membrane went to a *"dry bone"* (unspecified) whose secondary echoes were picked up by an even drier membrane and sent to the brain. One has to admit that with a generous if fanciful imagination this could well be interpreted as transduction through the middle ear - especially in birds. It is perhaps therefore a shame that Aristotle (384-322 BC), who was not only a doctor but also the son of a doctor, should have seemingly spoiled things. He was aware of the middle ear cleft and so incorporated that into the theory, saying that the air within the middle ear carried the echoes to the *heart*.[102] [103] He never rated the brain very highly, being of the opinion that it produced phlegm to prevent overheating of the body by the *"heart-furnace"*. Of course medicine as a whole was very cardio-centric in those days. Aristotle dissected the ears of a number of animals and described the pharyngo-tympanic tube, which was named after Eustachius.[104] This seems a little unfair to your authors. It was around the same period that Alcmaeon and Empodocles were writing in Greece that, Herodotus was describing the customs of the Egyptians. These included therapy using a variety of bizzarre substances to be placed in the ears. Much of our knowledge comes from the Ebers Papyrus[105] and it seems that in those days there was a high degree of specialisation in which one priest might treat deafness, another running ears.

Pythagoras investigated the physics of sound, noting that cords of different pitch were produced when a blacksmith struck the same anvil with hammers of different weight. He also managed to construct a simple scale using different lengths of string.[106]

Early in the third century BC the seat of medical interest moved to Alexandria where it remained until the first century AD. Unfortunately its medical library was burned down during the war against Julius Caesar and its contributions to medicine mostly lost. Gradually medical influence shifted, along with political and military power, to Rome.

There, Celsus wrote a medical encyclopaedia in the first century AD entitled *De Medicina* covering a whole range of medical subjects and rivalled only by those of Galen. Galen was a Greek physician who settled in Rome and who dominated medical thought from the second century AD for the next thirteen hundred years up until the time of Vesalius and the Renaissance. We now turn to this period.

The practice of dissection appears to have arisen first in Bologna towards·the end of the thirteenth century, and to have developed from the post-mortem examination which was ordered in cases of death under suspicious circumstances. The first anatomical textbook was the Anathomia of Mondino de Luzzi (Mundinus), written in 1316. As the entire process of dissection was completed within four days, this allowed little time for such refinements as the structure of the ear or throat. One of the most distinguished pupils of Mondino at Bologna was the French surgeon Guy de Chauliac (1300-1367) who may have been the first to use an ear speculum. However, it was Andreas Vesalius (1514-64) who truly reformed anatomy by the publication of his great work *De Humani corporis fabrica*. Some of his magnificent woodcuts have been attributed to Titian (1477-1576) and certainly Titian painted a portrait of Vesalius, now in the Pitti Palace. Appointed to the Chair of Anatomy at Padua whilst still in his twenties, he set himself to describe what he actually saw. To him we owe the names *atlas, vertebra, choanae* and *mitral valve*. He was the first to give an accurate description of the malleus and incus - the stapes was unknown until Ingrassia of Naples discovered it a few years later. He compared the malleus to a femur and the incus to a molar tooth.

Eustachius' book *Epistola de Auditus Organis* appeared in 1562 whilst he was working at the University of Rome and at the height of his fame. It is probably the earliest work to deal exclusively with the ear.[107] The structure which bears his name was known to the Greeks and, as has been said, was mentioned by Aristotle. Nevertheless, Eustachius was one of the first to accurately describe its structure, course and relations. Despite dividing it into bony and cartilaginous parts, the latter lined by mucous membrane, he compared it to a quill, thus once again demonstrating the flights of fancy and imagination shown by many of the latin races. Fallopius (1523-62), in describing the passage known as the *aqueduct of Fallopius* (the facial canal), stated that he gave it that name from its resemblance to a water pipe. He succeeded Vesalius at Padua and it is to him we are indebted for such names as *cochlea, labyrinth, velum palati* and *tympanum*. He also described and named the *chorda tympani*, the *trigeminal nerve*, the *auditory nerve* and the *glossopharyngeal nerve*. He was not only an anatomist but also a surgeon, leaving on record his treatment of aural polypus by means of destroying the growth with sulphuric acid, after the external auditory meatus had been protected by a lead tube.[108] Volcher Coiter (1534-1600), a Dutchman from Groningen was one of Fallopius' pupils and his work *De auditus instrumento* might be regarded as one of the first textbooks of otology. He became medical officer to the town of Nuremberg (long before it was made famous for the Nazi war crimes trials). Not only was he the first to study comparative anatomy on a large scale, but he also gave an account of the current views regarding the physiology of hearing. These were that the main function of the tympanic membrane was to protect the middle ear and preserve the purity of the contained air (aer implantus). The sound was conducted by this "implanted air" to the cochlea, which also contained air and acted like a resonator to increase the sound before it impinged on the auditory nerve. When one considers some of the essays handed in by medical students and nurses (in the days before multiple choice questionnaires and computer marking had been discovered), this is not bad for someone writing in the sixteenth century, and a Dutchman at that.

Another pupil of Fallopius was Fabricius (1537-1619), known as Fabricius ab Acquapendente, from his birthplace of Acquapendente, in a similar manner to Trevor from Bradford, who supplied the recreational videos for the Postgraduate Medical Officer Course at Sandhurst one of the authors was obliged to attend[w]. Anyway, Fabricius described in his book why the ears are situated on the head, why the pinna faces forwards and why its upper part is the broader and not movable. He eventually succeeded to the Chair of Anatomy and Surgery at Padua, but not before another of Fabricius' pupils, Julius Casserius (1561-1616) who took over from him in 1604. Amongst his pupils was William Harvey.

Learning Point
There were lots of important anatomists during the Renaissance, most of them working in Italy.

We now turn to the seventeenth-century. Probably the greatest book concerned with our subject to be produced in the seventeenth century and what is also generally accepted to be the first monograph to be published on the subject of otology was *Traité de l'Organe*

---

[w]

The reader should note that the much hyped video *Debbie Does Dallas* has very little to do with American football and even less to do with the city of Dallas.

de l'Ouïe.[109] This was published in 1683 by Duverney at the age of thirty-five and intended to be one of a series of books dealing with all the sensory organs. This was a new departure in medical writing in that it was written in his native French rather than Latin, although it was translated into Latin, German (1732) and English (1748), with twelve editions or translations being issued by 1750, twenty years after his death.[110] The words of the preface bear repeating:

Although I do not pretend that this work is entirely perfect, I hope at least, that the reader may here find something which has not been already described.

Your authors hope that the same holds true for this work. He corrected an age-old error by stating that the Eustachian tube was not an avenue of breathing or of hearing but was simply the channel through which the air of the tympanum was renewed; he also correctly explained the mechanism of bone conduction. This book was the first to contain an accurate account of the structure, function and diseases of the ear as opposed to pure anatomical description, although his anatomic drawings of the cochlea and middle ear are classics. He also reported that postmortem examinations of children had shown pus in the middle ear without infection in the brain, thus changing the two-thousand-year held belief that this is where discharge from the ear originated.

The next noteworthy contribution was made by someone whose name is, allegedly, now a household word. Presumably this is in households (such as those of your authors) where little else other than this subject is spoken. Valsalva (Antonio to his friends) lived from 1665-1723, thus just being in time for the Great Plague and the Fire of London, though was of course Italian (see *Learning Point*). After dissecting more than a thousand heads he wrote a treatise entitled *Tractatus de Aure Humana*, published in 1704 at Bologna[x], where he had long been a pupil of Malpighi, whom he succeeded in the Chair of Anatomy in 1697. It was he who divided the ear into three parts after studying *Caesar's Gallic Wars* at school[y], the outer, middle and inner ear. He applied the term *labyrinth* to the entire inner ear and suggested the use of the terms *scala vestibuli* and *scala tympani*. It is said that Valsalva was the first to examine the tympanic membrane in the living, but

---

[x] We are indebted to our military nursing officer colleague Major Stevie Webster for reminding us that within Italy Bologna is known as *Citta di Pompino* (Blow-job City).

[y] There is absolutely no evidence for this whatsoever.

in doing so he perpetuated the error of mistaking the notch of Rivinus for a foramen. This error was current among anatomists even before Rivinus of Leipzig published his thesis in 1717. His name is best remembered by the manouevre he described to force air to pass along the Eustachian tube (which he named in honour of Eustachius), originally describing it as a means of expelling pus in cases of otitis.

It comes as something of a relief to be able to describe an Englishman's contribution to what the reader might be in danger of assuming had become a subject dominated by foreigners. It would be wrong to assume that every Englishman was busy conquering, civilising and helping to paint a little more of the globe red[z]. Not only was William Harvey (1587-1657) producing his monumental work on the circulation of the blood, but Willis (1621-1675), who described the seventh and eight cranial nerves, devoted a chapter of his book to a discussion of hearing. His theory was that the tympanic membrane was set in motion by sounds and the vibrations thus produced transferred to the inner ear and auditory nerve. He also described a deaf woman he had observed who heard speech better in a noisy environment, a phenomenon now known as *Paracusia Willisiana.*

The eighteenth-century saw the development of the tuning fork by John Shaw (1711). Valsalva developed his manoeuvre to relieve negative pressure in the middle ear and instituted the correlation between clinical symptoms and postmortem findings.[111] Cotugno (1736-1822) discovered the fluids of the inner ear and described the fibres of the basilar membrane. He also proposed one of the first scientific theories of hearing.

It was not until the nineteenth-century that interest in otologic pathology, physiology and surgery, together with a rapid development in scientific understanding, all came together to promote rapid strides forward in our subject. Flourens, of Paris, published in 1828 his discovery of the action of the semi-circular canals and suggested that the acoustic nerve had two branches, one for hearing and one for balance.[112] Breuer of Vienna reported his experiments on rotated animals in 1874 and may have discovered nystagmus; his

---

[z]

A historical allusion to the fact that traditionally atlases &c had the British Empire shaded in red, a fact now not so obvious to the modern-day school child (known in educational circles as a *schoolkid*).

work later influenced Bárány in his research on the human vestibular system. In 1861 Prosper Menière reported his famous case of the girl who developed vertigo, nausea and tinnitus during a fatal illness, describing the changes found in the semi-circular canals at autopsy.[113] Prosper was a personal chum of both Victor Hugo and Balzac. He was not only a prolific botanist and archaeologist but was charming, witty and had bags of style; it's difficult to think of him as being French at all. He also published books on Greek and Latin poetry, in stark contrast to many of your modern medical Johnnies who think Ovid means "something to so with eggs". From humble beginnings he became the registrar of the notorious Baron Dupuytren at the Hôtel Dieu[aa], but really rose to fame when the Froggy government nominated him to ascertain whether or not the Duchesse de Barry was "with child". Menière's affirmation of her gravid state had a negative effect on the succession to the French throne but a positive influence on his own professional career! In the following year he was appointed to the Imperial Institution for Deaf Mutes and it was here that he became famous. His great service to medicine in general was to draw attention to the association of the labyrinth with balance, as hitherto dizzy spells had been ascribed to apoplexy or epilepsy. His famous case concerned a young lady who had arrived in Paris, having just travelled from Rheims "outside" (i.e. on top of[bb]) a stagecoach. She developed terrible vertigo, deafness, tinnitus and nystagmus and died shortly afterwards. Menière dissected her temporal bone and found a blood-stained perilymph (no mean feat for the 1860s!) which led him to further studies culminating in his statement:

> *There is every reason to believe that the essential lesion causing these symptoms lies in the semi-circular canals*

It was Prosper Menière's son Emile who first ascribed the disease named after his father to a vascular origin[114] (if one excludes the proponents of the apoplexy school). It is therefore a little ironic that there are historians who think that the diagnosis in the *mademoiselle* was almost certainly a leukaemic infiltration of the temporal bone. Your

---

[aa]

Which for the benefit of American and Australian readers was not a guest house but a hospital.

[bb]

The authors, who both used to go to school in Yorkshire on buses, well remember being asked "are you going inside or upstairs? long after open air top decks were obsolete.

authors do not number themselves amongst them, nor do they knowingly know anyone personally who holds such views, but would understand the reasons which might lead to such an opinion being given credence. Were either to find himself in Paris, as indeed one author was, briefly in 1991, the pursuance of such a conundrum would be low on their list of priorities. Of far more importance is the interesting derivation of the word *labyrinth*, which comes from the word for a double-headed axe, as any scholar of Greek or itinerant lumberjack holidaying in Greece will know. *Laburhinthos* did come to mean *maze*, but it seems that the Greeks got the word for the famous Cretan maze built by Daedalus under the palace of King Minos to house the fabulous minotaur[cc]. Another suggestion is the famous puzzle garden of the Egyptian 12th dynasty pharaoh, *Labyris*, at Crocodilopolis.

It was from such beginnings that our understanding of the vestibular system arose, a more detailed description of which the reader will meet in the section devoted specifically to this subject, if his patience will allow him to stay his curiosity for a little while longer whilst we finish the more general historical overview. In 1851, Corti, an Italian anatomist working in Würzburg, published his studies on the organ that now bears his name.[115]

In the latter half of the nineteenth century the scene shifts to Austria and Germany. The interest in diagnostic testing appears to have started with Weber in Leipzig where in 1825 he published his work on hearing testing with tuning forks and described what was later called the *Weber Test*. In 1855 Rinne in Göttingen reported his test and in 1855 Schwabach wrote an article criticizing both these tests and advocating his own.

The most influential person of this period was Politzer (1835-1920) who after studies in England, France and Germany was appointed Professor of Otology in Vienna in 1870. This cosmopolitan education was not unusual in those times, but one wonders whether anybody trying to emulate this today would be able to achieve enough backers in any one place to get anywhere at all. He was the first to photograph the tympanic membrane and his great textbook *Lehrbuch der Ohrenheilkunde* was translated into many languages and went through several editions. Helmholtz was initially trained as a

---

[cc]

We perhaps ought to explain for our international readers that the emblem of the Royal House of Minos was of course a double-headed axe or *laburos*.

military surgeon and then, after studying physiology at the University of Berlin and holding appointments in this subject at the Universities of Konigsburg and Heidelburg, was made professor of physics at Berlin in 1870. His tonal theory was published in 1863.[116]

(b) Noise Induced Hearing Loss.

Historical literature, even dating as far back as the Bible, is full of references to the harmful effects to the hearing of exposure to loud sounds over a prolonged period. Temporary threshold shift was described by Francis Bacon (1561-1626) in his *Sylva Sylvarum*. Many other references are often quoted, ranging from Alexander the Great's huge War Bell to Quasimodo. Perhaps worthy of mention is the fact that Chang and Eng Bunker, the original Siamese twins (1811-1874), had noise-induced hearing loss in opposite ears as a result of indulging their favourite hobby of rifle shooting. Eng fired from his right shoulder and Chang from his left; each suffered from deafness in the opposite ear. In contrast to writings on Quasimodo, which rarely contain a pure tone audiogram, this has been well documented. This cannot be said for the temporary threshold shift experienced by Admiral Rodney after firing eighty broadsides from HMS Invincible at the Froggy fleet in 1872.[117] Some might consider this a small price to pay for so much fun, unlike the poor unnamed officer who suffered permanent deafness after having his pinna too close to a cannon discharged at our traditional enemy during the Battle of Copenhagen in 1801. It is also averred that Admiral (then Captain) Hardy was deafened by cannonade on HMS Victory during the fateful Battle of Trafalgar; others firmly hold that this was a psychogenic loss which came on seconds before Lord Nelson's demise, and was feigned just so that he did not have to give the Admiral of the Fleet a kiss! This scurrilous suggestion is obviously made by those ignorant of the fact that the dying Sea Lord didn't in fact say *"Kiss Me! Hardy"* but *"Kismet[dd], Hardy!"* This is of course far more likely; Nelson was no queen and would hardly have been asking his comrade in arms for a kiss. In fact, even to this day there are no homosexuals to be found

---

[dd] Kismet: the fulfilment of destiny from the Turkish *gismet* - the lot. Evidently the Arabs often say *qismat*, expressing resignation to the Will of Allah. According to Lady Nelson, her husband was given to using this strange expression. Lady Hamilton's views on the subject are not recorded.

in the Armed Services as it is prohibited - as of course is alcoholism.

Much of the following is drawn from an article entitled *Downgraded Through My Hearing? Doctor* published by one of the authors in what is known as "The House Journal Of The Army", *The British Army Review*.[118] The authors are grateful to the editor not only for publishing it, not only for paying a fee, but also for allowing us to reproduce parts of it here, thus once again irritating our RAMC colleagues.

One of the earliest scientific studies was that of 1886 when Thomas Barr drew attention to the dangers to the hearing faced by boilermakers by the noise in their work.[119] The harmful effects of industrial noise exposure are thus well known, with Bunch publishing in 1937 the first audiometric data demonstrating the typical high frequency loss.[120] It might come as a surprise to those claimants who are constantly assailing us (especially the authors in their military practice) armed with the cry "But of course in those days there weren't such things as ear protectors - nobody knew anything about it in those days" to find that, shortly after the Second World War, efforts were being made to investigate the problems of industrial noise exposure. In America, the American Academy of Ophthalmology and Otolaryngology established in 1946 a special subcommittee *Noise in Industry* and this published the *Guide for Conservation of Hearing in Noise* which was used for the establishment of industrial hearing conservation programmes.[121] The reader is probably at this stage wondering why the authors have apparently taken leave of their senses and are talking about North America in a manner somewhat less than derogatory. Is the faint promise of a job (and enough money to make him as rich as Croesus) made to one of the authors turning his mind? Of course not! The diligent reader who has progressed as far as this knows better than that; he will also have a shrewd idea that the Yankee will usually have been pipped to the post by a matter of a few decades by an Englishman. For those poor souls bogged down in the mire of AIDS counselling and domestic trials, and hence unfamiliar with the 1911 work of Fleet Surgeon G G Borrett, we reproduce some of his writing:

> *In June 1911 the Admiralty issued lamb's wool to the Second Battle Squadron for trial....I was myself so convinced of the suitability of lamb's wool for protection against gun blast that I have continued its use up to the present date, giving it for trial and opinion to officers and men whenever gun fire has taken place, with the result that I still consider it the most suitable all-round form of ear protector yet suggested.[122]*

Thus, from over a hundred years ago there has been the acknowledgment that exposure to noise is detrimental to the sense of hearing, and steps have been taken to protect those at risk. At the outbreak of the First World War, Jobson Horne (1865-1953) was writing to the *Lancet*, which published 15 August 1914 a paper by him entitled *Gun Deafness And its Prevention*,[123] showing how quickly the profession was alerting itself and brothers in other specialties to the consequences of the ensuing conflict with regard to hearing. The cooperation shown by medical journals in this regard must be acknowledged, and was reinforced during the recent conflict in the Gulf when one of the authors managed to have reported in the *British Medical Journal* events as they were occurring at the Front[124] and an analysis of surgical operations performed within a few months of the successful conclusion of business.[125] Unwitting testimony as to how it was well-known that noise exposure caused deafness at the outbreak of War is given by the unusually named Mr Marriage[ee]:

> *Concussion deafness may be due to the constant noise of the guns firing day after day, or to the explosion in the immediate neighbourhood of the patient of a shell containing high explosive. In the former case, the results are similar to those seen in peace time in naval gunnery officers and boiler-makers, and in my experience a slight amount of permanent deafnes usually persists if the patients have been frequently exposed to the noise for long periods. The deafness due to the explosion of a shell is generally for a short time very severe, and at times the patient has been rendered unconscious, but as far as I know the deafness has never been absolute.*[126]

With the increased concern shown for deafness incurred under active service in contrast to the supreme indifference shown by the Victorian army, it was perhaps inevitable that there would be description of cases of non-organic hearing loss. These were dealt with in the typical robust manner current in the military medical services of the time.[ff] We reproduce the advice given by Colonel Birkett CB, to the Royal Society of Medicine:

> *As to the physical cases, they are, perhaps, the most pathetic we have to deal with. These men are broken in spirit, and their nerves are entirely shattered, and*

[ee]

Our international readers should take note that he was <u>not</u> the originator of the *marriage* ceremony.

[ff]

Thank goodness nothing like that could ever happen nowadays.

this condition is nearly always associated with mutism. It is, therefore, impossible to get any accurate results from our test. We begin by encouraging these men to hear and speak. Often, however, those methods do not succeed, and then we try to shame the men out of their disability before their companions-in-arms. Sometimes those means are successful. One method was letting off an alarm apparatus suddenly: this shocked one man so much that he eventually heard.[127]

At the same meeting Dundas Grant drew attention to an observation that sensory stimulation will cause dilatation of the pupil. His method was to contract the pupil with light and then blow a whistle, *"or in an extreme case, a motor-car hooter behind the patient"*, and watch for dilatation.

Within a few months of the outbreak of hostilities, the *British Medical Journal* was carrying articles about the relative merits of various ear defenders[128] and these were followed by a flurry of claims by various correspondents. One of these, in extolling the merits of the *Mallock-Armstrong* ear defender recounted his brother's opinion that *"They are splendid"* and that *"a section commander took one out of his ears and got a nasty surprise with the gun firing; he says he could not have believed that the difference would be so great"*.[129] The address of the supplier followed. As is so often the case in life, one tackles a problem with a fair degree of success, only to find that one's very means of so doing have precipitated a further problem. This was the case with an early form of ear defender made from celluloid, which, the Section of Otology of the Royal Society of Medicine was told: "should never be used, as on one ship during a battle several men had their ears damaged by the flash of a shell setting fire to the celluloid plugs which they wore".[130]

Sadly, the problem, with becoming commonplace, began to lose some of the impetus which had characterised the early stages of the War. By 1917 we are reading of "normal gun-deafness". In an article of such a title, T B Jobson theorised: *"that it would be of some interest and use to find out what proportion of soldiers exposed to gun-fire go deaf, to measure, as far as possible, the amount such deafness produced in a previously healthy ear (his emphasis), to ascertain whether this deafness is temporary or permanent, and to investigate the type of deafness so produced"*.[131]

The reader of nervous sensibilities may be reassured that he did not precipitate deafness in his subjects (more of that later), but examined patients who were in hospital for various wounds - *"the patients examined were Germans, and I must say they proved very intelligent subjects"*. He noted that over 80% did not consider themselves to have any hardness of hearing, but in none did he find perfect hearing. He concluded that:

> *Gun-deafness is of a very definite type - a mixed obstructive and nerve deafness. The amount of deafness as shown by a C2 fork is about -10 seconds aerial conduction and -4 seconds of bone conduction.*

A point of further interest to those who have some knowledge of the subject and who have learnt the traditional teaching (of which the authors are not terribly convinced) that the left ear of infantrymen becomes damaged is that Jobson found that the *right* ear was deafer than the left in the majority of cases. Perhaps it was because they were continentals. One of the authors, who spent three attachments working in the ENT departments of German military hospitals, has noticed that not only do they drive on the other side of the road, but the head mirror is worn over the *left* eye and the bull's eye lamp placed behind the patient's *right* shoulder. What a strange and wonderful world we live in.

Of course, nowadays the use of hearing protectors is an accepted practice in noisy industries and workers are usually protected by legislation which ensures that when ambient noise levels exceed 90dB the employer is obliged to provide approved protection and instruction in its use.[132] NIHL is classed as an industrial disease and, with the onus of proving negligence resting on the plaintiff, an action for damages can be brought. The purpose is to compensate for lack of earning ability rather than for injury sustained. In fact the Factory Inspectorate considered in 1906 that something that did not stop the worker working required no compensation. A successful action must demonstrate that the employer had a duty to take care and was negligent *"omitting to exercise the degree of care necessary in the circumstances"*. Damages can also be paid when ear defenders are provided but not used by the plaintiff, as was demonstrated by a High Court action.[133] Finally it must be shown that injury or damage was sustained during the employment. The time when the problem is first drawn to the employer's attention is an important factor in the amount of compensation payable. 1963 was a turning point in that it became a "date of knowledge" when an employer might reasonably be aware of the inherent risks and so negligence (and compensation) is backdated to then. An exception is made for British Rail, as the risks were documented by an industrial doctor in its employ in 1955 and so British Rail is liable from that date.

Despite the multitude of historical examples, anybody who is reviewing the problem of noise-induced hearing loss will be surprised at how little has been done to prevent its occurrence. It is a shame that Sir Hugh Cairns busied himself so much with neurosurgery, for as a consultant to the Army during the Second World War (with the rank of Brigadier), he made compulsory the wearing of motorcycle crash helmets.[134] The advice to use ear defenders was, alas, many years in coming.[135] Despite this, the Services have always been in the forefront of NIHL, primarily because it is such an important problem for them. Nevertheless fame can be shortlived. Squadron Leader Denis Lister Chadwick is recorded as writing the authoritative reference on this subject for that bible of ENT, Scott Brown's *Diseases of the Ear, Nose and Throat*.[136] It only lasted for that edition, though his untimely death may have spoiled his chances of a revision; this is not always the case though. Sir St Clair Thomson's book went on for a futher five years after his death. Denis always kept an interest in NIHL and often told the story of how his colleague Dr Vernon Knudson of UCLA (Authors' note: for once our American readers will know what is meant by this; it is added for the benefit of anyone from NW England that this refers to the University of California Los Angeles and not to the United Co-operative Laundry Association, with which it is often confused) had just published that noise damage was a definite hazard of loud modern music and discotheques. He went on to say that formal balls where the ladies wore long frocks and the windows were draped with heavy curtains were less hazardous because of the noise-damping effects of the fabrics. Quick to get hold of the muddy end of the wand, the tabloid newspapers responded a few days afterwards with the headlines:

MINISKIRTS CAUSE DEAFNESS

and

MINISKIRTS HARD ON THE EAR

Squadron Leader Denis Chadwick's work was continued within the Forces by E D D Dickson (1895-1979), who rose to the rank of Air Vice Marshall (equivalent to a two-star general), and who, in the words of his obituarist *"conducted during his service much important work on the effects of noise on hearing based not only on laboratory studies but also on field data"*.[137] He doesn't appear to have published any of it, however!

The problems of biological variation in sensitivity to noise make any form of prediction or calculation difficult, but the extent of the problem is illustrated by experiments performed in the 1940's on "medical student volunteers". These consisted of exposure of the unprotected ear 23cm to the left and 3.8cm in front of a rifle muzzle.

By performing audiograms between shots it was possible to *"compare the effects of similar exposure in different subjects, the variation in effect in the same subject when similar exposures were repeated, the effect of various rates of fire, and the development of deafness in relation to the number of rounds fired"*.[138] By these means the wide variation in human sensitivity was proven, and also the fact that in some subjects the deafness produced lasted up to three weeks!

The history of study of *how* noise causes deafness also goes back a long way. During the First World War, J S Fraser and John Fraser (a captain in the RAMC) realised that apart from the more gross changes which were often seen such as rupture of the membranous labyrinth and haemorrhages, the noise may *"destroy the delicate nerve endings in the cochlea"* (their emphasis). They go on to describe how

> *some observers hold that the change is a biochemical one, while others believe that it is of a molecular nature. Theodore has microscopically examined one case of labyrinth concussion followed by total deafness, and found a condition of degenerative neuritis similar to that described by Manase and Wittmaack in old people......microcopic examination of the ears from cases of shell deafness, which die from other causes years after the injury, would be of great value in clearing up the pathology of the condition, and especially in throwing light on the question of "degenerative neuritis" of the cochlea apparatus.*[139]

A stimulus was given to military consideration of this problem in 1973 when attention was drawn to the fact that the verdict at a recent court case had been that *"audiometric monitoring is part of the care expected of a responsible employer with workers exposed to hazardous levels of noise"*[140] and that a situation would arise whereby naval dockyard civilians would be treated differently from their Royal Navy counterparts and the Services were in danger of lagging behind in the responsibilities of employers as envisaged by the 1972 Government Code of Practice.[141] Furthermore, with no pre-enlistment audiogram there was no medico-legal defence to any claim for pre-existing hearing loss.

(c) Education of the Deaf.

The earliest recorded descriptions of the plight of the deaf are found in the Hebrew laws of biblical times, where it was stated that those who were deaf and had no speech were denied all legal rights. The Justinian Code ruled that the deaf without speech should be classified with lunatics and were without legal rights or obligations. The coupling of deafness with lunacy tended to be seen until the twentieth century. Thomas Braidwood (1715-1806) opened the first school for the deaf in 1766,[142] however John Bulwer (1614-1684) already knew and had published in 1648 in his *Philocophus, or the Deafe and Dumbe Man's Friend* that deaf mutes could be taught to lip read.[143] This was taken further by George Dalgarno (1626-1687) who advocated a one-handed manual alphabet to facilitate teaching the deaf to read and write in his publication *The Deaf and Dumb Man's Tutor*.[144] Sir Kenelm Digby, a 17th century corsair who established his reputation in a Levantine sea fight was interested in a wide range of medical and paramedical matters, the most interesting of which from our point of view concerns his meeting Bonet, one of the earliest teachers of the deaf in Madrid. This is described in his *Treatise Concerning Bodies*, published in 1664, where he gives an accurate description of the speech of the deaf and so helped stimulate the early English interest in their education.[145]

This century, Alexander Ewing (1896-1980) together with his wife Irene, developed the use of the new hearing aids which were being pioneered in the 1930s in the oral/aural philosophy in education of the deaf. In 1944 he was appointed director of the department of Education of the Deaf at the University of Manchester.[146]

(d) Vertigo.

The earliest description of what has come to be known as Menière's disorder came with the writings of Galen and his contemporary, Archigenes of Apamea.[147] Galen referred to the fact that these attacks could be provoked by a turning movement, and also when the *"head had been overheated for any other reason"*. This may be considered the earliest reference to emotional factors as a precipitating cause.[148]

Erasmus Darwin (1731-1802) developed the concept of evolution, which may have sparked off the interest shown by his grandson Charles. He devised a classification for vertigo which he described in detail in his Zoonomia. In this work he described the phenomenon of noise-induced vertigo (later to be known as *Tullio's phenomenon*) and also vertigo associated with tinnitus and hearing loss. He was one of the first to use electrotherapy in the treatment of vertigo, utilising Volta piles almost as soon as they had been described.[149]

In 1906 in Vienna, Bárány reported what was to become the first part of his monumental work on the vestibular system.[150] He received the Nobel Prize in 1914 for this and completed his work in Upsala in Sweden following the interruption of the First World War. It was his attempts in 1911 to create a fistula to decompress the labyrinth (for he was a clinical otologist, despite devoting most of his time to laboratory work) which led to the experiments of Jenkins in 1913[151] and Holmgren in Stockholm in 1918 to create a fistula into a semi-circular canal. Portmann was also stimulated by Bárány's studies on vertigo and in 1926 in Bordeaux reported a surgical decompression of the endolymphatic sac.[152]

Dandy in Baltimore reported the relief of symptoms from Menière's disease by section of the eighth nerve,[153] later revising the operation so as to include only the vestibular portion of the nerve in order to preserve hearing.[154] Owing to the technical difficulties involved this did no become widely used, although Dandy himself successfuly performed the operation on more than four hundred patients.

Techniques for labyrinthectomy were described by Schuknecht in 1956[155] and by Cawthorne in 1957.[156] Meanwhile Arslan was reporting the use of ultrasound to achieve the same purpose.[157] However it was not until 1938 that Sir Hugh Cairns published with C S Hallpike the classic paper confirming the long-suspected view that endolymphatic hydrops was associated with Menière's disease.[158]

(e) The Science of Audiometry.

Sir Astley Cooper insisted, by performing bone conduction tests with a watch held between the teeth, that the nerves of hearing be *"tolerably healthy"* before performing myringotomy, otherwise *"no alteration in the state of the membrane would be to any avail"*.[159]Unfortunately this advice was not always heeded and the operation fell into disrepute and into the hands of quacks. Francis Galton (1822-1911), who is probably better known for the fact that he was grandson of Erasmus Darwin and cousin to Charles Darwin, had, amongst his many interests, concern for hearing. The *Galton whistle*, which he developed, was used for many years to define the upper limits of hearing. He also performed pioneering work in the field of fingerprints and his biography is appropriately entitled *Francis Galton - The Life and Work of a Victorian Genius*.[160]

Thomas Buchanan (1782-1853) noted the effect of distance upon harmony and was perceptive enough to realise that:

> The Highland bagpipe, which at a little distance on a wide and blooming heath
> has a melody and sweetness particularly agreeable to the Scottish ear, may
> produce a stunning effect when played in a small apartment.[161]

Such sophistication was beyond the Glaswegian paediatric otolaryngologist who habitually banged the tuning fork upon the head of his young patients prior to performing the tuning fork tests as described by Weber and Rinne. Rinne himself never mentioned *positive* and *negative* forms of his test; this honour must go to Bezold.[162] It is interesting to know, however, than in Rinne's original description of his test he applied the tuning fork first to the incisor teeth and then to the mastoid process afterwards.[163] It is remarkable how often the name of Rinne is spelt by young medical people with an acute accent on the ee, as if he were French. They are only to be pitied for not realising that Friedrich Heinrich Adolf Rinne, Professor of Otolaryngology, University of Göttingen was not French at all, but German. He certainly did not use any form of accent - acute, grave or circumflex. Prosper Menière has also caused difficulties in this respect. In his manuscripts he utilised a grave accent on the second ee, but on his gravestone this appears as an acute. We considered recording this in the section on professional rivalries but we have no evidence that the stonemason had any personal animosity towards Prosper. Young people often compensate for this sleight by giving him both acute and grave accents on the first and second "e"s respectively. No doubt they mean well.

Alexander Grahan Bell became, like his father, a teacher in phonetics. This background was to serve him well when he came to develop the telephone (1876), which led later to such developments as the audiometer and hearing aid.[164] James Blyth developed what appears to have been the earliest audiometer made in the British Isles using a double telephone earpiece and altering the sound intensity by changing the number of resistances.[165]

An indication of what was in current usage for the measurement of hearing loss at the time of the first World War, when there was a tremendous increase in noise induced hearing loss, can be found from Sydney Scott's description of the test he used:

> With regard to the hearing test there are three features I think we should consider.
> The first is the determnination of the "tone-range"; the second of "tone-acuity";
> and the third "tone-analysis". The first is measured by forks and the monochord,
> which is far superior to Galton's whistle.[166] "Tone-acuity", for a given tone or

group of tones of known intensity is recorded by the distance limit of hearing a watch or acoumeter. Under "tone-analysis" will come the faculty of hearing the voice as whisper or in conversation.[167]

Basic research in our specialty was, towards the end of the nineteenth century, being carried out less by clinicians and more by scientists dedicated to pure research, as exemplified by the work of Helmholtz. This type of investigation was accelerated in the twentieth century by the development of the electric vacuum tube which made it possible for electic potentials never detected before to be studied. Alexander Ewing acquired in 1928 one of the earliest valve audiometers. He went on to develop conditioning testing for the testing of hearing in children and was later knighted for his work with the deaf.[168] The vacuum tube also made possible the development of the first modern clinical audiometer by the Western Electric Company, putting on a proper footing the experimental models developed by Hartman in 1878 and Hughes in 1879. This vacuum tube audiometer provided, for the first time, an instrument capable of making precise, recordable measurements throughout the auditory range.

In 1937 the cochlear potential was described by Wever and Bray in the experimental pyschology laboratory in Princeton, opening a totally new approach[169] which was further developed in laboratories throughout America and Europe. Békésy, a former engineer for the Hungarian telephone system, pursued his theories on hearing in Sweden and in 1941 was awarded a Nobel Prize.[170]

The first clinical measurement of acoustic impedance was by Metz in 1946.[171] In 1947, Békésy introduced his technique for semi-automatic audiometry which found not only application in standard threshold determination but also helping to determine the site of the lesion.[172] Ten years later, in 1957, Carhart added the tone decay test to the site of lesion test battery.[173]

(f) The World of Hearing Aids.

J H Curtis was responsible for the development of one of the early *Acoustical Chairs* and was also involved in work on ear trumpets.[174] A few years ago, the Portuguese ambassador to her Britannic Majesty offered Amplivox Ltd a very large sum of money for the State Throne of King Joao IV of Portugal. The company turned down the offer and the throne still stands in the Amplivox offices in Liverpool.[175] Why, one may ask, does Amplivox want to keep a Portuguese State Throne? The answer lies on the open lions' mouths at the end of the chair arms; in them are cleverly concealed ear trumpets, or acoustic hearing aids as they should more properly be designated. It seems a very elaborate way (even for a monarch) to conceal the fact that he was hard of hearing. The throne was British made, by the aforementioned J H Curtis, who pioneered the development of not only acoustical chairs but also other non-electrical hearing aids. Queen Victoria had one, and more recently Sir Winston Churchill. One of the authors (JRY, who lives in Devon) has prescribed an acoustic hearing aid as recently as 1990! Country folk "afeared on electrical gadgets" are more ready to accept them:there are no valves to break, no batteries or tubing problems and no difficult switches or volume controls with which arthritic old fingers must fumble. Distortion is minimal and, as one points it where one wants, background noise is cut down. Or, as one would say now, "signal to noise ratio is high".

The first electric hearing aid was made in 1872 by Alexander Graham Bell for his mother. He is described in Britannica as a Scottish-born audiologist best known as the inventor of the telephone. The early models were huge contraptions pushed around on wheels. It is interesting to note that the *Radioear* vacuum tube aid is monaural. One cannot help but feel that an optician who only dispensed monocles, telling his poor-sighted clients to forget about their other eye, would not maintain his credibility for very long. Many maintain that monaurality was either a function of cost (the parsimonious National Health Service cutting its expenses by half by only giving out one) or cosmetic stigma - on the grounds that it was bad enough having to wear one aid, let alone two. Neither of these considerations could have applied with Alexander's (he only adopted the name *Graham* when he was eleven) mother.

Carbon hearing aids preceded valves. They were so-called because they depended on fifty little graphite balls which changed their capacitance as sound passed through. Although very good for conductive deafness, owing to the constant low frequency background noise from the rattling balls, those suffering from sensori-neural hearing loss found them difficult to tolerate. This might have helped the still prevalent misconception that aids are only suitable for conductive deafness. Another problem which the carbon aids were susceptible to was a limited effective life, for as the balls rattled they became less spherical.

Transistors were invented in 1947 and transistorised aids came onto the market in the 1950s. They were easily camouflaged as hairslides, brooches and spectacles, though not as *Sony Walkmans*, which were not invented until the 1980s. By 1960 the National Health Service had caught up and the new improved aid, available to a limited number of selected individuals, used a transistor.

Hearing dogs for the deaf have been another way in which the problems of the hard of hearing have been alleviated. An advantage of an animal is the intense pleasure and satisfaction which can result and which is (usually) impossible with an inert piece of plastic. The system of training dogs was started in America and the news brought back to England in 1979 though it is contended that, like so many other things, it had all been done before in Germany at the end of the last century. Nevertheless, many people are now benefitting from the help of a dog trained to act as their ears and alert them when, for example, the telephone rings[gg]. Part of the training and reinforcement process is that whenever this is done, the dog should be rewarded with a sweet (or canine equivalent) and fulsome praise. Thus when one telephones the owner the first words one always hears are:

Good boy, well done!

which can be a little confusing or misleading for those unaware of this.[176] Nobody who owns and has read this book will fall into this trap.

Not all technological advances are real improvements. An ageing dowager newly equipped with an "in the ear" hearing aid found to her distress at a cocktail party that her aid had fallen out whilst she leant over to reach for some "nibbles". She spent the rest of the evening trying to fit a succession of peanuts into her ear.

[gg]

Hearing Dogs For The Deaf. Registered Charity No 293358 (England). London Road, Lewknor OXFORD OX9 5RY.

OTOLOGY

In which the authors explore the world of otology, paying particular attention to:

(a) The Early Development of the Subject

(b) The History of the Eustachian Catheter

(c) Artificial Perforation of the Tympanic Membrane

(d) The Discovery of Otosclerosis and Treatments with which it has been Tackled

(e) The Early History of the Mastoid Operation

(f) Acoustic Neuroma - the Magic and Romance Behind this Fascinating Tumour

(a) The Early Development of the Subject.

Hippocrates back in about 400 BC apparently inspected the tympanic membrane and observed that discharging ears were common in children whilst adults suffered from deafness. Some of his otologic writings were erroneous, for example he believed that otorrhoea was actually a fluid formed in the brain that discharged through the ear, but he became so revered that his conclusions were not challenged until the sixteenth century.[177] Possibly one of his greatest contributions was to free medicine from religious control and make it possible for men of scientific interest to make a contribution.

The Greek physician to the Emperor Trajan, Archigenes (98-117 AD), devised a novel, if drastic cure for deafness: he blew a trumpet into the patient's ear.[178] He was presumably working on the basic premise of utilising any residual salvageable hearing. At about the same time as this, Celsus was trying to treat deaf mutes by pulling out the tongue *"with pluckers"* and cutting the membrane beneath.[179] This was based on the tale told by Herodotus about the dumb son of Croesus, the fabulously rich king of Lydia, who suddenly spoke after breaking his tongue tie through terror when an enemy soldier was on the point of slaying his father. Ethical committees are loathe to grant licences to repeat this experiment. Archigenes' treatment did, however, live on for some time. In the seventeenth century Bonet reported a *"new improved method"*:

> This defect some have tried to remedy by taking the deaf into the country and
> into valleys where the voice has a greater resonance, and there making them
> utter loud sounds, and with such violence that blood issued from their mouths;
> also by placing them in barrels where their voice re-echoed, and where being
> more closely imprisoned, they might hear it.

By the beginning of the first-century AD, Rome had become the centre for medical thought. It was here that Celsus wrote a medical encyclopaedia entitled *De Medicina* in which he stated that otitis media could lead to insanity. He also prescribed the use of vinegar instilled into the ear to kill insects before attempting their removal from the external canal. The following thirteen centuries were dominated by the writings of a Greek who settled in Rome, Galen. He was a prolific writer, producing more than ninety volumes on a variety of medical topics, based on his close observation of diseases and dissections and also influenced by the writings of Hippocrates. It was he who suggested draining the mastoid in the presence of acute infections, but as far as is known he never attempted the operation.

74

(b) The History of the Eustachian Catheter.

Archibald Cleland (1700-1771) was the first British practitioner to describe Eustachian tube catheterisation but his purpose was to irrigate the middle ear with warm water or simply to blow air in it in order to *"dilate the tube sufficiently for discharge of excrementitious matter"*.[180] The Eustachian catheter has something in common with the laryngoscope - both have been designed by non-medical people in Paris. Apart from that they have nothing in common. Before the eighteenth century the treatment of deafness and diseases of the ear was entirely empiric, despite the advances of the anatomists. In 1724 a postmaster at Versailles named Deme-Gilles Guyot succeeded in relieving his own deafness by the use of a curved tube passed into the mouth and behind the palate. Perhaps his own description to the Academe Royale des Sciences de Paris best conveys his thoughts:

> *La pièce principale en est un tuyau recourbé, que l'on insinué au fond de la bouche derrière et au-dessus du palais, à dessein de l'appliquer au pavillon de la trompe qu'on veut injecter. On en lave au moins l'embouchure, ce qui peut être utile en certain case.*[181]

One wonders how many postmen these days could write something like this, but unfortunately it excited little comment, the anatomists of the day being unconvinced that one could syringe out the Eustachian tube by way of the mouth. No further progress was made until 1741 when a Scottish military surgeon, Archibald Cleland, of General Wade's Regiment of Horse recommended, independently, the same procedure:

> *The passage should be lubricated by throwing a little warm water into it by a syringe fixed to a silver tube which is introduced through the nose into the oval opening of the duct at the posterior part of the nares...The pipes of the syringe are made small, of silver, to admit of bending them, as occasion offers, and for the most part, resemble small catheters. They are mounted with a sheep's ureter, the other end of which is fixed to an ivory pipe which is fitted to the syringe, whereby warm water may be injected, or they will admit to blow into the Eustachian tube and so force air into the barrel of the ear and dilate the tube sufficiently for the discharge of excrementitious matter.*[182]

He also described a *"convex glass which will dart the collected rays [of sunlight] into the bottom of the ear"*. The Eustachian catheter was not only the first instrument to be commonly used for the treatment of deafness, but its mainstay. That is not to imply that everyone was adept at this - Thomas Buchanan was described by the German otologist Wilhelm Kramer (1801-1875) as *"the only English practitioner who understands and practices catheterism of the Eustachian tube"*.[183] The value of catheterisation was written up in 1871 by Peter Allen[184] and it is interesting to contrast the picture then with that pertaining a hundred years later when it had become obsolete and replaced by myringotomy with or without the placement of a ventilation tube - both of which would have been technically possible much earlier had the desire to do so been present.

(c) Artificial Perforation of the Tympanic Membrane.

William Cheselden (1688-1752) experimented on dogs to see if hearing was possible with a perforated tympanic membrane but as his results were inconclusive he tried to experiment on the human subject. It seems that even in those days ethical committees could be a hindrance but he managed to obtain permission to experiment on a condemned man who would receive a pardon if he submitted to it. This provoked such a fierce public outcry, especially as it was rumoured that the criminal was Cheselden's cousin, that it was abandoned.[185] It was not until Shrapnell investigated the minute structure of the tympanic membrane and proved that the so-called *foramen of Rivinus* did not exist[186] that perforation of the drum, the *myringotomy* could be put on a scientific basis. In 1760 a strolling quack named Eli punctured the eardrum to relieve deafness. This was repeated some forty years later by Sir Astley Cooper who gained the Copley Medal of the Royal Society in 1802 for doing the same thing. He had noted in 1800 in two of his patients that partial loss of the tympanic membrane caused only a slight hardness of hearing and not the total deafness which was popularly imagined. This, incidently, demonstrates that he had the ability not only to clearly see the drum but also to distinguish between total and subtotal perforations. The following year he suggested that *"the deafness which arises from an obstruction of the Eustachian tube"* might be treated by puncturing the eardrum. He did this, using *"a trochar and cannula, of the size of a common probe"* which he thrust through the antero-inferior part. As mentioned in our prolegomenon, he did not, however, pursue this *"as he was afraid to be thought an aurist"*.[187] This was not an unreasonable fear. Curtis read a paper at the Medical Society of London in 1837, to be followed by Joseph Toynbee, who was present, writing to the Lancet on the fallacies of his pathology and registering a vow that he would *"rescue aural surgery from the hands of quacks"*. Astley Cooper also recognised that Eustachian obstruction could arise from the common cold, the tonsils and fibrosis from venereal ulcers.[188] Within a short time a minute trephine known as the *Aurisector* was invented and used to punch out a tiny disc from the ear drum. Owing to the fact that the beneficial results tended to be transient, the operation, which was advised as a cure for deafness, was soon forgotten. The first to advise paracentesis in acute suppuration of the middle ear was John Cunningham Saunders (1773-1810),[189] the same man who founded, in 1805, Moorfields Hospital.

(d) The Discovery of Otosclerosis and the Treatments with which it has been Tackled.

It was Valsalva (1665-1723) who was the first to demonstrate the presence of ankylosis of the stapes at post mortem examinations:

> One day in the cadaver of a deaf person I found the cause of the deafness. The membrane covering the oval window was ossified in such a way that the base of the stapes and the periphery of the window formed a solid piece and the stapes had become immobile.[190]

More than a century was to pass before the significance of this was to become apparent. In 1877, Kessel reported that he had succeeded in mobilising the stapes through the tympanic membrane. Later he removed the stapes and replaced it with a membrane for the successful relief of otosclerotic deafness.[191] Mobilisation of the stapes was reported from France in 1890 by Camille Miot (1838-1904) and in the year of his death he was considered as being most identified with this operation, *"which he practised and advocated with the strongest convictions as to its value"*.[192] In 1892, Jack of Boston reported the removal of the stapes with the relief of deafness in several patients. However these surgical procedures risked the serious dangers of infection, meningitis and death and so were not accepted for clinical usage by the otologists of the time.

Ballance reported in 1900 accidently opening the lateral semicircular canal during a petromastoidectomy. He covered the opening with a skin graft which not only arrested the vertigo but improved the patient's hearing.[193] This was taken further by Sourdille in France in 1932. Basing his work on suggestions made by Bárány and that done previously by Holmgren in making a fistula into the lateral semi-circular canal,[194] he managed to succeed in developing an effective two-stage operation for the relief of deafness from otosclerosis.[195] In the same year that Sourdille published his self-styled *new technique*,

Holmgren published *The Surgery of Otosclerosis.*[196]

In 1938, Lempert in New York reported his *fenestra novovalis* technique, a one-stage operation through an endaural approach for creating a semi-circular canal fistula.[197] This procedure was quickly accepted for clinical use, with Lempert undertaking to train many otologists to perform it. History can be vague as to the actual precedence. Dr Ion Simson Hall is recorded as being among the first otologists in the 1930s to develop and carry out the fenestration operation for the relief of otosclerotic deafness and to use magnification. He is also credited with immediately grasping the significance of stapedectomy "when it was introduced in the late 1950s" and he was considered by his obituarist to have become "one of the first European surgeons to forsake fenestration for a procedure that some still regarded as too experimental, but which soon became standard",[198] thus illustrating not only the value of a good obituary but the danger of basing too much historical study solely on such sources. This is reinforced when one reads how the obituarist of Sir Terence Cawthorne considered that he also was one of the first to adopt the fenestration operation.[199]

In 1952 Rosen in New York presented a paper describing the successful mobilisation of the stapes footplate after reflecting the tympanic membrane.[200] His *reintroduction* of this operation was made possible because of modern control of infection and the development of improved instrumentation and magnification. A few years later, in 1958, Shea in Memphis revived the stapedectomy,[201] which has now become the standard operative procedure for otoscerotic fixation of the stapes. It is interesting to see how what in retrospect is seen as merely a short step along the long road to the development of an answer to a clinical problem can be viewed by those with a special interest as being of monumental import. Sam Rosen, in his autobiography written in 1973 and comprising 268 pages devotes only the following few lines to stapedectomy:

> *Nevertheless, stapedectomy has proved of value. We have learned how to use a synthetic material called Gelfoam together with a prosthesis made of wire and Teflon in cases where removing the stapes entirely is the only way in which hearing can be restored. The combination usually results in the formation of a thin, flexible membrane across the opening of the oval window - a new, natural windowpane which holds in the perilymph but vibrates with the prosthetic stapes to conduct sound waves to the fluid and thence to the delicate apparatus of the nerves of hearing.*[202]

(e) The Early History of the Mastoid Operation.

Galen's surgical advice is strangely modern, when he states that carious bone should be removed after making an incision behind the ear.[203] However, Sir Charles Ballance, in his magnificent work *The Surgery of the Temporal Bone* states that the earliest suggestion of opening the mastoid by operation is found in the writings of the anatomist Johannes Riolanus (the younger) who suggested trephining the mastoid in 1649. This was for tinnitus, but he does not appear to have carried his suggestion into practice.[204] The Van Leyden engraving of 1524 (too familiar to us all to warrant any further reproduction) suggests that such surgery may have been practised even earlier, but in fact this may simply be a representation of the opening of a sebaceous cyst. It is considered that the first successful operation on the mastoid for the evacuation of pus was in 1774 by Jean Louis Petit (1674-1750). This was not simply the enlargement of a persistent fistulous track but a deliberate search for pus.[205] The Frenchman's effort was quickly followed in 1776 by Jasser, a Prussian army surgeon. Unfortunately, in the years that followed, this operation was used to treat tinnitus and a number of conditions not related to infection and hence fell into disrepute.

There were attempts at rehabilitation. In 1838, George Pilcher won the Fothergillian Gold Medal of the Medical Society of London for his work: *The Structure, Economy and Diseases of the Ear*. Toynbee was probably the most influential otologist of the nineteenth century and spent much of his professional life dissecting human temporal bones obtained at necropsy, achieving a collection of almost two thousand.[206] He published his observations and ideas for surgery in in 1860 in *Diseases of the Ear*, which became a classic amongst medical writings. Hinton, who was a colleague of Toynbee, discovered that aural polyps originated in the middle ear and also showed the fatal course of a cholesteatoma that led to meningitis and a brain abscess.[207]

Of course, for surgical advances to be made, there had to be concurrent developments in equipment. John Brunton (1836-1899) invented an otoscope comprising an eyepiece, convergent lens and side viewing arm.[208] Thomas Buchanan was one of the first to recommend the use of artificial light to better inspect the eardrum, calling his instrument his *Inspector Auris*. One of his reviewers commented that *"Hull was the very spot to give birth to such a substitute for solar light"*.[209]

It was the research of Sir Arbuthnot Lane which led to important advances in the treatment of inflammation of the middle ear and its complications. Prior to his work there had been no definite description of the mastoid antrum and suppuration had been dealt with by means of a small trephine. He demonstrated the inadequacy of such methods and devised chisels and gouges by which the antrum could be freely and rapidly explored, and it is claimed that he was the first in the United Kingdom to open the mastoid antrum [210]. His treatment of pyaemia resulting from inflammation of the middle ear is illustrated in the *Lancet* of 1893:

> *Out of six cases of pyaemia due to middle ear disease on which up to that time Lane had operated he had lost only one, and death arose in that case from an extension of the septic process along the petrosal to the cavernous sinuses.*[211]

Radical mastoidectomy was first performed in 1889 by Küster, whose technique has remained unaltered through the years. Dalby, the first aural surgeon at St George's Hospital, London advocated the value of mastoid surgery, but never performed it himself, allegedly because his age and training were against him - he was not of the new era of Listerian doctines. This did not handicap him unduly - twenty years after qualifying he was knighted (1886).[212] It is not known with certainty whether his low postoperative complication rate was the deciding factor. He certainly was very careful, being one of the first to advocate the use of a dental drill to remove exostoses from the external auditory meatus. These small pieces of bone have occupied a role in otology in disproportion to their clinical importance, having formed the doctoral thesis of another ENT knight, Professor Donald Harrison. It was perhaps somewhat unkindly pointed out in *Scott Brown's Otolaryngology*[213] that much work had been done prior to this, however, in that Van Gilse had been the first to demonstrate a higher incidence in cold water bathers.[214] E P Fowler Jnr and P M Osman, working with guinea pigs, were able to demonstrate the formation of new bone following cold water irrigation,[215] and, as is stated in the textbook:

> *Harrison*[216] *carried out similar experiments with guinea pigs and found histological evidence of new bone formation in the deep meatus.*

Michael Kersebaum[hh] draws attention to the fact that this condition was formerly known in Germany as *swimmers' ear*. This was in the time when swimming pools consisted of rectangular pits filled with chlorinated cold water and before the days of artificial palm trees, wave-making machines and warm water. It is now known there as *surfers' ear* as it is considered that it is only in those individuals exposed to the rigours of cold sea

---

[hh]

Contemporary

water that the condition occurs. Both authors have applied to go to Malibu to "hang ten" and test this hypothesis but as yet research funds have not been forthcoming.

The incision known by the name of *Wilde* belongs to the father of the well-known playwright, Oscar. At this point it should be noted that neither Wilde nor Toynbee ever performed a mastoidectomy. One of our colleagues[ii] was appalled to hear a fellow surgeon referring to a "Vild" incision. The poor fool was under the misapprehension that he came from Germany. When the reader learns that this occurred in Newcastle he will perhaps be a little more inclined to believe what we agree appears rather a tall story, but, we are assured, perfectly true. Sir William Wilde advocating penetrating the mastoid bone, but actually used his incision only for draining post-auricular abscesses. In 1853 he published a volume on aural surgery. He was not thought to be homosexual, but then again, in Newcastle, neither was his son.

An illustration as to how dangerous it could have been in the past to have any sort of serious infection is shown by an incident involving the remarkable Lt Colonel A D Wintle. He was admitted in the 1920s following a riding accident to a military hospital where he met a boy trumpeter by the name of Mays. He was in the part of the ward popularly known as the *Stiff's Retreat* suffering from mastoiditis and diphtheria, usually a fatal combination. Not put out in the least, he roared at him:

> *What's all this nonsense about dying, May? You know it is an offence for a Royal Dragoon to die in bed. You will stop dying at once, and when you get up - get your bloody hair cut.*[217]

May later confided that after that he was too terrified to die. Wintle was quite a fearsome self-assured character who did not suffer fools gladly, holding that:

> *There are essentially only two classes of Englishmen: those who believe themselves superior to foreigners - and those who know they are.*

His extreme patriotism stood him in good stead during the First World War when the man stood next to him in the trenches was blown to pieces. Whilst lesser men might have taken flight or panicked, he forced himself to stand to attention with the shells

---

[ii]

Lt Col J A J Deans FRCS RAMC, former Command Consultant Surgeon, British Army.

bursting around him *"until I was able to become again an Englishman of action"*. At Ypres he was blown up by a mine, lost one eye and much of the sight of the other, plus a kneecap, five and a half fingers and one and a half thumbs. Despite this he discharged himself from hospital, returned to the Front, captured thirty five prisoners single-handed and won the Military Cross. He died in 1966, his last wish being that the band of his old regiment, the Royal Dragoons, should play Schubert's *Serenade* at his funeral. Unfortunately it was serving overseas so ex-trumpeter Mays, fortified with a bottle of whisky, stood to attention at the funeral and *sang* the entire *Serenade* himself. But we are digressing. Whilst doing so, we may as well throw in the *British Medical Journal* editorial of 1902 which revealed that a Chicago surgeon had *"recently devised a procedure by which he hoped to transplant a healthy human ear, presumably to take the place of one destroyed by disease"*.[218] The enterprising otologist could not find any volunteers and had to advertise, offering \$300 (worth £60 at that time [ii]) to anyone willing to have their ears amputated. In doing so he would be, according to the first chapter of the first book of Blackstone's Commentaries, be guilty of the crime of *mayhem*. It is stated that

> *A man's limbs, by which for the present we only understand those members which may be useful to him in fight, and the loss of which alone amounts to mayhem by the Common Law, are also the gift of the wise Creator to enable to protect himself from external injuries in a state of nature.*

(f) The Acoustic Neuroma - The Magic and Romance behind this Fascinating Tumour.

The audiogram was unremarkable, as were tomograms of the petrous apex. Audiological investigations such as tone decay, speech etc were similarly inconclusive, with no abnormal interaural latency difference of waves J1-V on ABR; caloric testing showed no canal paresis. The woman, a timid, anxious -looking housewife of middle years sat impassively in front of me. I thought it best to be open with her.

> *I am afraid the tests we have performed so far have proved inconclusive. The next step is what has been termed the "gold standard".[219] It is magnetic resonance imaging with gadolinium enhancement, and has replaced computerized tomogram air meatography as the radiological investigation of choice due to its greater accuracy and lower morbidity.[220] You might like to think of it as a scan;*

[ii]

Of course, £60 was worth more than a round of drinks then.

it is quite painless.

She sat unmoved.

I've come about me Dad. His deaf aid's on the blink.

The above report was found in the case notes of a doctor admitted to a rest home for the incurably optimistic. He is making a good recovery and, having graduated from the basket-weaving course, is now working night and day in the metalwork department on what he calls a *holy grail.*

For those of our readers who have not read Eduard Sandifort's treatise of 1777 (incredible though this may seem, one of your authors had only just learnt of this seminal work, and had even then only read it in translation!) it will come as a surprise to learn that the salient features of the acoustic neuroma were well known to the eighteenth century neuro-otologist. Chapter 9 of his *Observationes Anatomico-Pathologicae* deals with a firm corpuscle adhering to the auditory nerve, or as he puts it *"de duro quodam corpusculo nervo auditorio adherente".*

He was quite thorough in his description, which for the benefit of our American and Australian readers, we reproduce in translation:

> *The position and firm adhesion of this growth clearly showed that it had compressed the auditory nerve; this was also proved by the depression visible in the medulla oblongata and the neighbouring soft tissue, and it was further confirmed by the extension of the tubercle into the foramen of the auditory nerve which was considerably diminished in size, and finally by a comparison of the right auditory nerve with the left.*[221]

MILITARY PROWESS WITHIN THE FIELD OF OTOLARYNGOLOGY

In which the authors venture into the martial exploits of famous otolaryngologists and recount how military adventures led to advances in the world of civilian otolaryngological practice &c &c.

MILITARY PROWESS WITHIN THE FIELD OF OTOLARYNGOLOGY

For those of our readers who have difficulty in retaining knowledge (even such interesting and important facts as to be found in these chapters) we remind you that the first British hospital specialising in otology was set up as a dispensary in Soho Square by J H Curtis (1778-1860) who began his professional life as a dispenser in the Royal Navy (see page 14).

Henry Jones Shrapnel (1761-1842) was a surgeon to the Royal South Gloucester Regiment of Light Infantry Militia who later married Edward Jenner's ward.[222] The exact relationship between the military and medical precedence of this illustrious name has exercised medical brains in a manner surpassed only by that other conundrum, the exact relationship between Bill Lund and Valerie Lund, Professor of Rhinology. The redoubtable Shrapnel went on to become a surgeon and anatomist in London and in former times the pars flaccida of the tympanic membrane used to be known by his name, a habit used now only by very old or eccentric otologists who show disdain for the modern Latin terminology. Strangely enough, the German for the military shrapnel is *das Schrapnell*, with an added "c" and the extra "l" at the end.[223] When it comes to the anatomical reference they witter on about *Shrapnell-Membran*, spelling the name more correctly, which goes to show what a funny world we live in. Worse, in the reference book we used, they had committed the error[kk] of thinking that the year of his death was 1841.[224] At this point we should perhaps point out a possible source of confusion which has no doubt been the source of endless problems for the British Army of the Rhine: *Der Granatapfel* is not the German for a type of munition such as a handgrenade (which is *die Hand Granate*), but is in fact a pomegranate.

Possibly in an attempt to compensate for such problems and minimise disruption the British military otolaryngological world has had a remarkable degree of stability. In the past forty years there have been only three different Consultant Advisors in this subject to the RAMC. The obituary of the first (1952-1969), Brigadier H N Perkins, reads:

[kk]

In examination terms this would probably not be considered a *lethal* mistake; except of course unless one of the authors was holding the position of examiner, a circumstance which is hardly ever likely to happen.

His peer group admired the near miracle whereby he remained in the same attractive posting for seventeen years in a service mostly characterised by three year postings.[225]

Edwin Arthur Peters (1868-1945) is chiefly remembered for his aural speculum but his other claim to fame is that he must have been one of the most aged junior officers to serve in the RAMC. He obtained the M.D.in 1900 and FRCS three years later and was appointed to the staff of the Royal Ear Hospital, which was subsequently amalgamated with University College Hospital. At the outbreak of the First World War he was 46 and was put in charge of the ENT department of one of the largest military hospitals, the Royal Victoria Hospital at Netley - with the rank of captain![226]

Sir James Dundas-Grant (1854-1946) served during the war as consultant to the King George Military Hospital *and numerous officer hospitals.*[227] By this is meant hospitals where all the patients were officers, and the nurses much prettier. He is best remembered for his love of inventing really useful instruments. Perhaps the best known is his antrum seeking probe. This was originally designed by the great man for identifying the aditus ad antrum in cortical mastoidectomies. The practical difficulty which it was designed to overcome was in differentiating the actual antrum from other mastoid cortex cells which may mimic it. The idea was to insert Jimmy's antrum seeker in the supposed antrum and then try to lift the skull vertically off the operating table. If the seeker is in the antrum then the whole weight of the head is supported and it rises. If, however, it is only a cell, then the bony septum will break under the strain as one tries to lift the head. For some unaccountable reason this indispensable aid to mastoidectomy is sometimes known as Dundas Grant's Incus Dislocator! The other cunning instrument which bears his name is the cold air caloric apparatus which is designed to blow ice-cold air into mastoid cavities or ears with perforations to see if the organ of balance is intact. He described during the First World War with pride how it had apparently been taken up by the Army otologist in France as a regular official test:

> *It is a tube of copper, covered with a little cotton moistened with ethyl chloride. A current of air is driven through it, and as soon as it is at its coldest, as tested on one's own cheek, the patient's head is thrown back at an angle fo 60 degrees and he is told to turn his eyes to the opposite side, when nystagmus should be produced in from 28 to 30 seconds.*[228]

He fails to mention that the coil rapidly becomes encrusted with ice, which, if it doesn't block up the main tube, causes frostbite of the finger skin of the operator which becomes stuck solid to the aural probe end of the instrument.

He is not the only military person to have had an inventive streak. Archibald Cleland (c1700-1771) secured a job as surgeon to General Wade's regiment, the 3rd Dragoon Guards, but during eight years saw no action and had plenty of time to develop several novel instruments; of course things are quite different now. Amongst these, which he demonstrated to the Royal Society, were a candle-powered illuminator for inspecting eardrums and an ivory vacuum tube for sucking them back out after they had been forced in from the blast of nearby explosions.[229] Presumably his failure to see any active service prevented him managing to test this in the field.

A story of note regarding British phlegm in the face of adversity worth recounting concerns the famous Lt Col A D Wintle, about whose attitude to the sick the reader has already learnt much (see page 81). He was captured in France during the Second World War whilst working as an undercover agent, managed to escape but was recaptured. At this stage he decided that his Vichy French guards looked too scruffy and threatened to go on hunger strike if they did not smarten up. Such was his power that they cleaned their buttons, polished their boots and promised to shave every day.[230] It is fortunate that in the twentieth-century the treatment of prisoners of war, although in many instances such as were found in the Far East during the Second World War where conditions were incredibibly harsh, has not matched that meted out in Ancient Times. For example, in 1300 BC the Pharoah Menphtha inscibed on the walls the following inventory to commemorate his victory over Libyan invaders: *Phalluses cut off Libyans: 6,359 (6 from generals), from Siculians 222, Etruscans and Greeks, 542. Grand total of phalluses brought to the king 6,111.*[231] This is not the origin of the word *dictator*, but it has been considered by many as one of the earliest examples of surgical audit. But the audit cycle was not completed, blah, blah, blah.

Sir Harold Gillies, who can be considered the "father" of plastic surgery began his career as an otolaryngologist. His new specialty was founded in 1916, born as part of the preparations of the RAMC for the battle of the Somme and due almost entirely to the work of Major Gillies, working under his consultant Sir Wm Arbuthnot Lane.[232] It has been often noted that under the driving force of war and war conditions, advances in medicine can be made which would take much longer to occur in peacetime.[233] Nevertheless, you would have thought they would have made him an acting Lieutenant

Colonel. Still, Robert Jones was only a captain, and Gordon-Taylor had already been on the staff of the Middlesex Hospital for seven years when, at the beginning of the 1914 war, he was commissioned into the RAMC at the age of thirty-six. The end of the war found him Consultant Surgeon to the Fourth Army - with the rank of major![234] A fuller account of the development of plastic surgery and its relationship to war can be found in Antony Wallace's[ll] excellent monograph.[235] Whilst on the subject of plastic surgery we should record a story not covered by Mr Wallace concerning Robin McNab Jones who once had otolaryngological responsibilities for, among other places, Her Majesty's Prison Wormwood Scrubs. He had just agreed to perform a rhinoplasty on one particularly belligerent, twisted-nosed convict (so that after his reforming penal servitude, he could face a new life with a new nose) when the warder, who strictly speaking should not disclose what the prisoner was doing time for, confided that he was imprisoned for shooting the plastic surgeon who had done his first rhinoplasty.

The specialty has not been short of heroes. William Tyler Gardiner (1889-1938) was commissioned into the Royal Army Medical Corps during the First World War from the staff of the Ear and Throat Department of the Royal Infirmary of Edinburgh and subsequently won the Military Cross.[236] Josephine Collier (1894-1972) served as a specialist otologist in the Second World War with the Royal Army Medical Corps in the rank of major.[237] She did not remain behind at home in a garrison hospital but saw service both in North Africa and Italy with Monty's 8th Army where the use of specialists far forward up near the frontline was pioneered.[238]

E D D Dickson, who retired from the Royal Air Force as an Air Vice Marshal after much work on noise induced hearing loss, did much work with the Royal National Institute for the Deaf, becoming its chairman from 1960 to 1971 and President from 1975 until his death in 1979.[239] Ross Coles[mm] reminds us of the need for education of the

---

[ll]

Contemporary; a stalwart of the Military Surgical Society, this plastic surgeon of note has, since retirement, worked tirelessly in the field of medical history and is to be found twice a week cataloguing he muniments of St Bartholomew's hospital. He has also provided endless support and encouragement for JDCB.

[mm]

Ross Coles liked the life of a National Serviceman in the Royal Navy so much that he stayed on for seventeen years, retiring as a Surgeon Commander. Two of these years

fighting man regarding the value of good hearing and, equally, the danger in which he could be placed through failing to appreciate this. This was brought home forcibly to the Royal Marines in Aden. A patrol lying in ambush came under fire from rebel tribesmen when their position was given away through the noise of a marine urinating from a kneeling position instead of remaining lying down as he had been ordered. (This reminds the authors of one of their comrades in arms in the Territorial Army who, in order to pass water from the comfort of his camp bed, used a snooker cue holder pushed through the door flaps of his tent as an "extension" [nn].) It was as a result of the need to impress the value of good hearing and the dangers of making unnecessary noise that Ross was asked to make a training film for the Royal Navy and Royal Marines. He decided to replicate the Aden incident and a suitable Geordie Royal Marine was primed with several pints of beer. A mock ambush position was set up on a cold starlit night in January in England and, as the cameras rolled, he relieved himself. So well had he prepared himself in the pub beforehand that the very expensive film had all but been used up before he had finished and he was surrounded by clouds of steam. Nevertheless, the sound levels had been tuned and it was a "take". But Royal Marines are nothing if not enthusiastic. Turning full (face) to the cameras he grinned broadly and asked: *"Di'ye wanna fart as weel?"*.

Another amusing incident Ross recounts from his service with the Royal Navy was when he was measuring the noise hazard from mortars at the Royal Military College of Science, Shrivenham. One practice bomb landed in the centre of the Army cricket pitch.[oo] There were no fatalities but the grass suffered severe contusions as did the Army

---

were in an unusual appointment for a doctor - as the Queen's sailing master in charge of the Royal sailing yachts. He then became Senior Research Fellow, later Professor, in audiology at Southampton University and finally Deputy-Director at the Medical Research Council Institute of Hearing Research in Nottingham. When this was first being penned, he was President of the Section of Otology, Royal Society of Medicine.

[nn]

The late Major Jack Roberts went away for his two week annual camp with the Territorial Army in 1939 to return several years later after the successful conclusion of the Second World War. A stalwart of 207 (Manchester) General Hospital Royal Army Medical Corps (Volunteers), he was only allowed to resign eight years after the normal retirement age.

[oo]

For our American readers, this is a game totally beyond the comprehension of not only many foreigners but most women. Lasting up to several days, its chief purpose seems to be to get the master of the house out of the way whilst spring cleaning etc is undertaken.

groundsman's regard for an officer of a sister service. Some years earlier, he had been no luckier with a hand grenade at Port Said when, as assistant officer of the watch, he had to throw grenades over the side, six per hour at irregular intervals, to deter possible frogman attacks. Unfortunately, unbeknown to Ross, a destroyer had come alongside and one of the grenades exploded on its deck. The subsequent enquiry determined that medical officers were not to be entrusted with such weaponry.

Much has been made of the advances which the wily can make to their medical career by a sojourn in the Forces, especially during wartime and contacts made have proved, to many, invaluable in later life. The converse is of course also true. Joseph Lister, as a Quaker, did not go to the Crimea, the only one of the seven residents in his year in the infirmary who did not. His surgical chief, Richard James Mackenzie (1821-1857) went to the war but did not come back, dying of asiatic cholera at Sebastopol. Had he returned it is doubtful if Lister would have ever got his staff appointment.[240]

RHINOLOGY

In which the authors consider the following topics:

(a) The History of Rhinoplasty

(b) The History of Nasal Polyps and their Removal

(c) The Tragedy of Benjamin Babington and his Forgotten Disease

(d) Other Interesting Pickings

(a) The History of Rhinoplasty.

Professor Gaspare Tagliacozzi published his surgical textbook in Bologna in 1597 in which he described in great detail and with beautiful illustrations how the nose could be reconstructed by means of a flap from the inner surface of the upper arm. This was the so-called *"Italian Rhinoplasty"*, a technique which had been invented earlier that century by a Sicilian peasant, Antonio Branca.[241] It would be wrong to think that this was the first mention of the operation of rhinoplasty, however, for writing in Varanasi (Benares) in about 600 BC Susruta Samhita devoted the sixteenth chapter of his surgical textbook to "The techniques of ear puncture and plastic surgery".[242] The *"Indian Rhinoplasty"* was referred to by a British Army staff surgeon working in Madras in his contribution to the *Gentleman's Magazine* in 1794.[243] It consisted of a flap from the centre of the forehead based on the supratrochlear vessels being dropped downwards to reconstruct the nose. Certain families of the brick-maker class had been practising the technique since 1000 AD, no doubt being given plenty of trade by the fact that amputation of the nose was often used as a punishment.[244] It was of utmost importance for these foreign chaps to restore the nose as accurately as posible, and with two nostrils, for these are indispensible for anyone who practises Hatha yoga. The left and right nostrils coexist as complementary pathways which allow *"prana"* to enter the body with each breath. *Prana*, the subtle life force, flows through channels in the astral body, known as the *"nadis"*. The left nostril is the pathway of the *nadi* called *"ida"*, and the right nostril is the path of *"pingala"*.[245] Neither of your authors have knowingly practised Hatha yoga, though one made the acquaintance of a woman in Berlin who as part of her stage act wrapped her legs around in a manner similar to the "lotus" position whilst practising some deep breathing exercises.

(b) The History of Nasal Polyps and their Removal.

The sponge method which Hippocrates employed to remove nasal polypi was practised by rhinologists certainly as late as the eighties of the nineteenth-century and probably even later - it is mentioned in Voltolini's textbook in 1888. The ends of three or four strings were tied to a sponge cut to the proper size and shape, and the other ends knotted together were fastened to the eye of a soft malleable tin or lead probe which was pushed through the nose into the pharynx. The ends of the strings were passed over the end of a forked probe held in the pharynx and by traction against this the sponge was dragged into the pharynx, bringing the polypi with it. Paul of Aegina was the last of the Byzantine compilers and a physician of high repute practising in Alexandria until his death in AD 690. He advised that a knotted cord be introduced into the nose and passed out by way of the palate and mouth. Then, *"drawing it with both hands, we saw away, as it were, with the knots the fleshy bodies..."*.[246] Fallopius was, amongst his many other achievements, also an important figure in rhinology, for he invented the the wire snare for the removal of nasal polypi. Notice how he does not give too many specific technical details away:

> *I take a silver tube which is neither too broad nor too narrow, then a brass or other metal wire, sufficiently thick, preferably the iron wire from which harpsicords are made. This doubled I place in the tube, so that from this wire a loop is made at one end of the tube by which, used in the nares, I remove the polypi.*[247]

(c) The Tragedy of Benjamin Babington and his Forgotten Disease.

Osler Weber Rendu disease should more properly be known under the name of Benjamin Babington who was appointed to the staff of Guy's Hospital in 1837. In this he was perhaps aided by his parents who took the precaution of giving him the middle name of Guy to commemorate his birth in the building. He qualified in medicine from the University of Cambridge at the relatively late age of thirty-one following service in the Royal Navy and the East India Company. He is also considered to be the inventor of the laryngoscope, or as he called it the *"glottiscope"*. Hodgkin referred to it as the *speculum laryngis*. It was Babington who first described hereditary haemorrhagic telangiectasia, in 1865, noting the condition in five consecutive generations of one family.[248] However many others took to describing the condition later:- Rendu in 1896, Osler in 1901 and Weber in 1907 and these names are commonly associated with it. His achievement is all the more notable for the fact that at the time he was writing this up hereditary disease was, except in the most general terms, unknown in clinical medicine. Mendel's work of 1867 lay buried until the turn of the century and it was not until the early 1900s that the terms *dominant* and *recessive* inheritance were applied, following the work of Archibald Garrod. A pretender to the crown of discoverer of hereditary haemorrhagic telangiectasia is H Gawen Sutton who wrote in the *Medical Mirror*.[249] His claim however depends on one short paragraph:

That epistaxis is hereditary on some families has been asserted by so many physicians that is would be difficult not to believe that it is so; but if careful enquiry is made into the medical history of different families it will readily be seen that such is really the case.

Your authors feel confident that the reader will agree with us that this claim can be dismissed.

(d) Other Interesting Pickings.

The problem of epistaxis has led to a variety of methods to assuage the flow being devised. One of the more unusual which your authors were able to find was the advice given in the *British Medical Journal* of 1876 that *"if the case be slight, simple means often succeed, such as the application of a bag of ice to the testicles or to the breasts"*.[250]

The first to discuss deviations of the nasal septum appears to have been Quelmaltz who published a treatise on this subject in 1750 entitled *Programma de Narium earumque Septi Incurvatione*. He considered the causes to be pressure upon the nose during difficult labour, falls in infancy, continually pushing the finger into the nose in childhood, and inflammatory conditions. Morgagni, in his *De Sedibus et Causis Morborum* also describes spurs and deviations of the septum which he considered to be due to *"the too rapid growth of the septum relative to the other bones of the upper jaw, from which reason there necessarily results a curvature"*. At a meeting of the laryngological section of the Royal Society of Medicine in 1913, H A Fisch introduced his rhinometer as *"an instrument designed for the purpose of ascertaining whether slight degrees of nasal obstruction are present"*.[251] The principle of the instrument lay in measuring the distance through which a column of water could be moved in a definite time and it consisted of a glass tube with a wide nose-piece and a resistance at the distal end. At the demonstration a member of the audience vouched for its efficacy in that he had exposed a case of a girl claiming under the Workmen's Compensation Act. Following an accident in a mill where her nasal bones had been smashed and the septum crumpled she had claimed that she suffered from nasal obstruction. With the aid of the rhinomanometer he could demonstrate that following straightening of the septum and removal of the turbinal bodies performed by a colleague *"there was even more than the normal amount of airway"*.

Edward Baber not only reviewed the operation of adenoidectomy but devised a special bandage which when wound from the top of the head under the chin would correct the habit of mouth breathing.[252] It cannot be said with any certainty whether the fashion amongst certain ladies including current royalty for wearing headsquares in such a manner dates from this. He also designed a nasal speculum in 1881.

A 1952 copy of the *British Medical Journal* contains in its section *Any Questions?* delightful unwitting testimony as to the role of patients, and particularly women, in society. The question posed is what advice should be given to an adult nose-picker (the age and sex are not specified). Readers are advised thus:

> *Long-ingrained habits are exceedingly difficult to treat, and the possibility of success depends almost wholly on the determination of the patient to win his freedom. In this case one is led to wonder why treatment is now being sought at this very late date. Has the patient, long contented with his habit, had some change in his life which has altered his attitude? He might, for instance, have become engaged or married to a woman who objects strongly to his habit and is pressing for treatment.......Pyschotherapy might possibly be considered, but does not look hopeful.*[253]

John Bostock (1773-1846) was the first to describe hay fever or allergic rhinitis (1819) which he named *summer catarrh*.[254]

The maxillary sinus was first described in 1651 by Nathaniel Highmore (1613-85) following a case of suppuration in the antrum. This was caused by an abscess of a canine tooth. Following its removal, the patient thrust a silver bodkin into the empty socket and *"was exceedingly frightened to find it pass, as it did, almost to her eyes. And upon further trial with a small feather stripped of its plume, was so terrified as to consult the Doctor and others about it, imagining nothing less than it had gone to her brain".*[255] What had actually happened was that the feather had doubled up in the antrum. William Cowper (1666-1709) was a little bolder. Writing in his chapter on diseases of the nose in Drake's *Anthropologia Nova* (1707) he describes an operation to release pus in acute sinusitis. His method was to approach the maxillary antrum by removing the first molar tooth and then allow drainage via the mouth.[256]

A cheap simple non-invasive test (and hence a sure-fire winner in any audit competition, had there been any in those days) for sinusitis was dark room illumination. Using a darkened room, an electic torch was place in the mouth, thus illuminating the paranasal sinuses. Peter McKelvie considers that this investigation has become less common since the demise of the custom whereby the nurses tended to be pretty young girls and doctors (real) men. The authors have not pursued this line of enquiry, considering it to be sexist.

SURGERY OF THE HEAD & NECK

In which the authors consider the following topics:

(a) The Case of the Gunner with the Silver Jaw

(b) The History of Tonsillectomy and some of the Instruments by which it can be Perfomed

(c) Some Famous Tracheostomies

(d) Milestones in the Development of Laryngology

(e) Some Highlights of Head and Neck Surgery

(a) The Case of the Gunner with the Silver Jaw.

Nowhere is the idea that war hastens the development, through necessity, of medical advances more aptly shown than in the case of the "gunner with the silver jaw". This concerns a French casualty during the siege of Antwerp in 1832 and was reported at the time in the *London Medical Gazette*.[257] A shell exploded nearby injuring his right forearm and the lower part of his face to such an extent that virtually all his mandible and the alveolar process and teeth of the left upper jaw and hard palate were destroyed. His medical attendant, Major Forjet took a plaster cast of the defect and commissioned the metal engraver and goldsmith Verschuylen of Antwerp to manufacture a prosthesis for him. It seems that the plaster cast and a prosthesis fitting it which are exhibited in the anatomical museum in Edinburgh refer to this case for it is known that Sir George Ballingall, who occupied the chair for military surgery there from 1823 to 1855 received such a thing from his friend the dentist Robert Nasmyth for him to use in demonstrations and bearing the words:

Inventé et fait par I P A Verschuylen, Orfèvre et Ciseleur à Anvers 1833

He subsequently made use of this in his writings.[258] From the *London Medical Gazette* description we find that the main part of the prosthesis was a facial half-mask to substitute for the lost lower face and it consisted of three functional components. There was an oval opening in the mouth region which could be covered with a silver sheet movable via an elastic spring hinge. Inside was an artificial mandible with alveolar process and complete dental arch plus an arch of the mouth which was fitted to the lower surface of the tongue. The mandible as well as the outer silver sheet could be flicked downward for food to be taken in without removing the whole mask. Also within was a basin to receive the secretions from the remaining mucous and salivary glands which could be drained through a small opening in the left chin area. The whole assembly was held in place with rubber straps and the use of oil paint and false whiskers ensured the best possible cosmetic result. When one compares the rather primitive surgery still being undertaken in those days, this stands out as quite a successful marriage of the art of the prosthesis maker coupled with surgical and physiological principles.

History does not relate whether the gunner with the silver jaw managed to retain all his functions within the maxillo-facial department, but your authors are reminded of the cautionary tale of Moira, related to them by Stevie Webster. The poor lady, sadly now dead, though not from this reason, was performing fellatio when she dislocated her temporo-mandibular joint. The treatment for this is to immediately reduce it by placing a finger in the mouth and clicking the offending jaw back into place. Unfortunately there was no room for a finger.

(b) The History of Tonsillectomy and some of the Instruments by which it can be Performed.

Next to circumcision, the operation of tonsillectomy is claimed as one of the oldest in surgery.[259] Celsus (53 BC - 7 AD) in *De Medicina*[260] gives the earliest description of tonsillectomy saying that indurated tonsils result from inflammation and as they are only covered by a thin membrane, can be removed by being separated with the finger nail. If this is not possible he advised that they should be grasped with a hook and excised with a bistoury. Unfortunately we are not told what his indications were, though with the inevitable progress of time its benefits were invoked for many diverse reasons. These ranged from masturbation to bedwetting (enuresis nocturna). Other evils which might be alleviated by adeno-tonsillectomy are night terrors, convulsions, laryngismus stridulus, twitching during sleep, chorea, petit mal, stammering, stuttering, asthma, vomiting, chronic bronchitis, defective chest expansion, dead voice, exophthalmic goitre,[261] rheumatism, affections of the heart, nephritis, latent tuberculosis, and an interesting condition in which the child complains of headaches, fatigue, listlessness and is peevish and bad-tempered; some cannot fix their attention on anything for any length of time, a condition termed *aprosexia* by Guye.[262] In addition to these can be added recurrent tonsillitis and ear infections.

Cheselden pre-empted the modern method of veterinary castration of farm animals in which the vet introduces a thick elastic band like a Dinky car tyre over the scrotum with a special introducer and then pushes it off proximal to the testes, which then slowly turn black like a couple of prunes and drop off into the field where they are considered a delicacy by crows and cats. (*Cuadrillos* or fighting bulls' balls are a Spanish hors d'oeuvre.) Anyway, Cheselden transfixed the lower tonsillar pole with a double-threaded needle which he tightened daily for a few days until they dropped off and the patient didn't need any breakfast.

One of the authors (JRY) was treated to the spectacle of guillotine tonsillectomy by Neville Winter (Bill) Gill. Before proceeding any further we should first of all clear up the widespread misunderstanding that the guillotine used in judicial execution was of French origin. At the time when such an instrument was first in use, the average Frenchman could not understand the workings of a wheelbarrow, let alone a complex piece of machinery such as a guillotine. It, of course, derives from Yorkshire. The aptly named Gibbet Street in Halifax bears witness to the fact that it was in this town and also Hull (giving rise to the expression "From Hull, Hell and Halifax, good Lord deliver us") that public executions took place on a regular basis. In Halifax a mechanical method of execution for the stealing of cloth was introduced by Norman barons and referred to in the Holinshead Chronicle of 1587 when *"felons were instantly beheaded with an engine"*. The practice ceased in 1650, since when the crime rate has escalated. The occasion for Gill to revert to this method of tonsillectomy was an attempt to reduce his waiting list and he considered that it would be quicker than using the dissection method. The first important point evidently about guillotining is that one has to have an anaesthetist who gives diethyl ether! This held unpleasant memories for JRY who remembered doing a house surgeon day-case list in Doncaster with a strange bleary-eyed Scottish lady anaesthetist who always insisted on using ether for everything. This was often unkindly attributed to her own predilection for the aroma of the gas, but this must have been wrong for your author always remembers her smelling strongly of Scotch whisky. Her colleagues in the anaesthetic department had hidden all the Schimmelbusch masks from her, but, undeterred, she had improvised her own substitute using gamgee. Her lists were especially memorable as they took place each Tuesday morning. This followed the only night off in the week allowed to JRY[pp]. In his rather precious state he did not really need the handicap of the coughing and spluttering during the irritative phase of the ether anaesthetic, which for some reason did not seem to affect the old Scot. It was with some relief that it was learnt that Bill Gill's anaesthetist, Dr Ian Gow, would be using a closed circuit and that the Glaswegian beldam had cruelly misled everybody. Working a bit like a Laurel and Hardy double act, the old anaesthetist put the child to sleep whilst NWG checked the springs on the guillotine and the theatre staff looked for ice. Most surgeons are used to hearing gas-passers say:

He's almost asleep, you can start now.

[pp]

In even earlier times they used to send children down the mines. In the opinion of one of the authors this would have been preferable to working as a house surgeon in Doncaster.

One was therefore a little taken aback on this occasion to hear him say, somewhat paradoxically:

You can start now Bill, he's almost woken up!

The position of the patient's head was also quite remarkable as it was over the head of the table and supported in mid-air by the anaesthetist who grasped the child's hair, unencumbered by such anaesthetic impediments as mask, bag or tubes. NWG moved in like a whippet, snipping out the two scampi-like organs and flicking them deftly over his shoulder with a skilful wrist action. One stuck to a tile on the theatre wall for a few seconds before plopping down to the floor; the other went down the top of the author's right Wellington. He was later advised as to the reason why older ENT surgeons pull their trouser bottoms outside their boots. Then, the only part of the melodrama clearly seen, he triumphantly held up a St Clair Thomson adenoid curette above his head like a poignard with the sad adenoids dangling, impaled on its three tines. But the show was not yet over! Peter the theatre sister, who always wore his theatre cap carefully ironed and shaped to look like an American sailor hat, rushed forward pushing a bucket on wheels. This contained large lumps of ice, water, and a sponge. Like an experienced boxing second (which he most assuredly was not), Bill Gill soaked up the icy water and then drenched the head of the now spluttering, coughing bairn, which was still being held by the hair, gripped like a macabre trophy by the anaesthetist. Peter (Hello Sailor) the sister then flung the child over his shoulder and carried him head hanging down to fling him onto a trolley in the "tonsil position" face down, buttocks upwards, Kama Sutra-like on a pile of pillows to be returned to the ward in a welter of blood, sweat, tears and iced water. Bill Gill in the meantime had snatched up his still-burning pipe which he used to leave between cases on the operating theatre window sill, much to Peter's chagrin, and began to puff furiously make sure that it was still alight. It was his firmly-held believe that if it had gone out then the operation had taken too long. Trevor Farrington, who was a senior registrar at the time looked at JRY, who was at that time senior house officer, and said:

And they say Music Hall is dead!

Whilst we are on the subject of guillotines, we would be remiss in not mentioning Dr Physick (not a fictional character but who actually lived, if this is not too extravagant a term, in Philadelphia 1786-1837) who modified Benjamin Bell's uvulotome. The more astute of our readers may wonder why Ben Bell was excising the uvula (which, incidently is the diminutive of the Latin *uva*, a grape; in the same manner that Nigel Lawson's daughter is called Nigella, a facility denied, or at least not wise, for any female offspring of, for example, Salman Rushdie to adopt; but we digress). What is perhaps even more surprising is that the Nigerians[qq] still perform uvulectomy on boys at puberty. It is not known why, but one theory is that they misinterpreted the message about circumcision. Like circumcision, it is a dicey business and fatalities are not unknown. It seems that Jewish Talmudic Law, with which some of our readers may be as unfamiliar as the authors, states that if a mother has lost two sons from post-circumcision haemorrhage, the third son does not have to be done. This, although going against strict Darwinian principles, seems entirely reasonable. In the same way that carcinoma of the foreskin is unknown in Jews, so carcinoma of the uvula is similarly rare amongst Nigerians, thus proving the great value of these two procedures.

The French surgeon Pierre Joseph Desault (1745-95) seems to have been the first to use a special instrument for the removal of tonsils. It was a modification of an instrument known as the *cystotome* or *kiotome*, which was used for dividing cysts of the bladder.[263] It consisted of a metallic sheath cut into the shape of a half-moon at one end across which a knife blade could pass after it had been adjusted to the tonsil which was drawn into it by means of a hook. It was not generally adopted, and in the words of the ENT historian Robert Scott Stevenson, *"eventually lapsed into desuetude"*.

Day-case tonsillectomy is not a new idea. The French (for what that's worth) have always done tonsillectomy as a day case and up to the 1940s and 50s in Great Britain the same applied. On most days outside the Manchester Ear Hospital at about tea-time, a sad queue of children would come down the steps and spit blood into the gutter while waiting for the tram home. This *may* have been the grounds for Ava Gardner's immortal words in Samuel Bronston's colourful epic *55 Days At Peking* when she comforts a wounded young soldier in hospital with the words
Go to sleep, soldier, and dream of Manchester.

He promptly died.

Of course, a large aspect of the management of operations such as tonsillectomy is cultural. It is almost unheard of <u>now</u> for tonsillectomy to be performed under local anaesthesia within Great Britain, yet quite commonplace in Germany. One of your authors (JDCB) had experience of this whilst attached to the Bundeswehr, providing a contrast

---

[qq]

From *Nigeria*, a country in Africa.

with the British Army where even antral washout is usually done under general anaesthesia[π]. The patient is placed in a sitting position with the operator in front of him. Local anaesthetic is injected by means of a very long needle and the bleeding points are tied off by means of a sling introduced with a *Roderbinder*. This has a ratchet mechanism by which the sling is tightened, the whole affair being, with practice, operated with one hand. Great care should be taken to avoid saying *"whoops"* whenever the instrument is misbehaving, as it tends to do in the first few dozen cases as this tends to put the patient off. An alternative we suggest is *"Now that is an interesting new development"*. In similar manner, no matter what disaster has occurred in virtually any operation the situation can often be retrieved by asking the medical students to step forward and take a closer look and sending for the photographer from the Medical Illustration Department. By the time he has arrived, it is a certainty that one of the students will have either fainted or touched something. The formidable Sir Arbuthnot Lane needed no recourse to methods such as these: he is reported as having in 1892 ligated the common carotid artery to stop haemorrhage following the removal of a tonsil. Intravenous saline was given and the patient recovered.[264]

The word *tonsil* comes from the Latin *tonsilla* which means "mooring post"; it is, of course, so abundantly obvious why the oro-pharyngeal tonsils should be compared to a nautical device on which to hitch one's boat, that we will not insult the dear reader's intelligence by dwelling on the subject. The Dutch, French, Germans, Italians, Portuguese and Spanish (listed in alphabetical order; normally we would put the French and Italians last) call them *amygdala* from the Greek word for almond, which clearly shows how devious the minds of Europeans can be, when the organs bear such a striking resemblance to bollards. The name *adenoids* (which organ was once known as *Luschka's Tonsil*[ss]) is

---

[π]

The unwary would be foolish to read too much into this as an interpretation of the fighting qualities of the respective soldiers as an examination of this century's world wars will show.

[ss]

After the German anatomist H. von Luschka (1820-75), the same man who described the holes in the IVth ventricle, the almost non-existent cartilages in the anterior part of the vocal cords and the infantile bursa of the pharynx, not to mention his gland whose function is unknown but it lies in front and below the tip of the coccyx. Were ever any of our readers to be confronted with a question needing his accomplishments to be listed we feel confident that in comparison with those poor students without this book and still in a state of darkness they would be extraordinarily well equipped.

a modern day contraction of the full term *adenoid vegetations* of the nasopharynx. The word adenoid is of course derived from the Greek *aden* .....meaning acorn.[265] Incidently, this makes one wonder how many words the Greeks had for this, since *balanos* also means acorn[266] and is not, as some believe, Greek for *policeman's helmet*. The German word for acorn is the same as that used by them for the glans penis though. Our American readers are advised to take a short break now.

(c) Some Famous Tracheostomies.

Although the first tracheotomy is attributed to Alexander the Great (356-323 BC) who is alleged to have pushed in the tip of his sword and then twisted it (just the tip, mind you!) into the trachea of one of his comrades in arms who was suffering obstruction from a war wound (unspecified) there is in fact little hard evidence for this as the great General was remarkably lax at writing up his cases.

Both Galen and Aretaeus refer to cutting the trachea, and Paul of Aegina has a chapter on "laryngotomy". Nothing more is heard of the operation until the Arab physicians Rhazes, Avicenna and Avenzoar each described it. Apparently none of them ever performed it. The best description is by Fabricius, who was the first to criticize the transverse skin incision employed up to his time and advised that it should be made vertically over the third and fourth tracheal cartilages. He also recommended the use of a small, straight and short cannula with two wings at its outer ends to prevent it from slipping into the trachea. Despite all this he also never performed it. Fortunately for him he did not have to fill out a book to show the Specialist Advisory Committee. Nor of course did any of the members of the Specialist Advisory Committee, but that is another story. The first person to actually perform the operation was Antonio Musa Brasavola (1490-1554), in 1546. The first appearance of the word *tracheotomy* is in the *Libri Chirurgiales Xll* of Thomas Fienus (1567-1631), Professor of Medicine at Louvain,[tt] which was published in 1649. The first person to perform tracheostomy in Britain was

---

[tt] Your authors were completely unaware of this fact when in 1979 during the free weekend of a Territorial Army exercise in Belgium they went on a motor-coach pub crawl which incorporated this town which is the home of the Stella Artois Brewery. Amazing isn't it?

George Martin (1702-43) of St Andrews. He was also the first to advise the use of a double tracheotomy tube.[267] J P O'Dwyer first introduced laryngeal intubation of respiratory obstruction in 1885.

(d) Milestones in the Development of Laryngology

Monteverdi, Handel, Gluck, Mozart and Rossini all wrote roles in their operas for male sopranos and such castrated singers often achieved wide and long-lasting acclaim; this might have proved some consolation. The most famous was Carlo Broschi (1705-1782) who was known as the *"Singer of Kings"*.[268] It seems that his vocal range extended from 128-1365 Hz and he could hold a note for 120 seconds. After his formal operatic career was over he was retained by the court of Phillipe V, King of Spain as an adviser. It is claimed that he was one of the first exponents of music therapy in that Phillipe's successor, Ferdinand VI, who suffered from melancholia resembling a form of schizophrenia found that the only therapy which had any effect was to listen to his singing. This continued each evening, with the same songs, for twenty years. It is strange what foreigners will get up to isn't it? Things haven't changed with time: it was reported that in Sicily the police arrested an otolaryngologist for operating on a Mafia boss's larynx. The reason for this was to alter his voice so that phone-tap evidence against him would be discredited.[269] Of course that sort of thing couldn't happen in Britain - for the criminal would need the tapes in order to sell his story and make his fortune from the tabloid newspapers.

John Avery may well have anticipated Garcia in 1848 with his instruments. He did not confine himself to the larynx but sought to examine various parts of the body including the urethra and bladder using a speculum and reflector. For the larynx he had a head mirror illuminated by candle light and a laryngeal mirror housed within a speculum. He was unable to fulfil his wish of photographing the view he obtained because patients would not tolerate the speculum for long enough and unfortunately he did not write up his results.[270] His claim can also be bettered, and this time with the support of Morell Mackenzie, who considered that the first laryngoscope was devised by Benjamin Babington. He demonstrated to the Hunterian Society his instrument for examining the larynx in 1829.[271] Who can tell what might have happened if there had been the annual prize for developing an instrument available in those days and he had entered. He probably wouldn't have won. In 1889 Voltolini was able to perform the first transoral illuminated laryngeal operation. However, before this, Sir Duncan Gibb (1821-1876) had made the first attempt in England to remove a growth from the larynx through laryngo-fissure in 1865,[272] a year after he wrote his book *On diseases of the throat and windpipe.*[273] A mere twenty-one years later, the Polish surgeon Mikulicz performed the first pharyngotomy for tumour (in 1886).

(e) Some Highlights of Head and Neck Surgery.

John Fothergill (1712-80), the famous wealthy Quaker physician, philanthropist, friend of the American colonists and botanists published his *Account of the Sore Throat attended with Ulcers* in 1748 and an account of what sounds a true diphtheria was written in 1757 by John Huxham (1692-1768).[274] He was the first to notice that diphtheria was sometimes followed by paralysis of the soft palate.

T B ("Tubby") Layton was an ENT surgeon appointed to the staff of Guy's Hospital in 1912. His time there was broken by service in the Great War 1914-1918, which in the 1920s came to be knwon as the First World War; it is now often abbreviated to WW1, but not in this book. He was twice mentioned in despatches and won the Distinguished Service Order, claiming to be the first British officer to enter Jerusalem when it was taken by Allenby's forces. His interest to us, apart from all that, is that he had an interesting case of Hereditary Haemorrhagic Telangiectasia on his books at Guy's and this woman became known over the years to virtually every department in the hospital. She was most grateful, however, during her long period of treatment of the cautery of a large telangiectasis in her mouth which was receiving trauma from her false teeth (Am: which was being traumatized by her dental prosthesis). Cautery was performed by the Professor of Surgery of the time, Ian McColl. She went so far as to say that it was the single most useful thing that had ever been done for her. Ian McColl was subsequently elevated to the peerage, though it is not clear whether it was solely as a result of this act of kindness.

One of the most epoch-making papers (in the opinion of Professor Grey Turner) was that by Arbuthnot Lane on the excision of a carcinoma of the cervical oesophagus, performed in 1909, in which the gap in the oesophagus was repaired with flaps of skin from the neck. Colledge tells us that it was this original operation which inspired Wilfred Trotter to devise similar operations for the excision of carcinomata of the pharynx.[275] Dr

Hardy Hendren, now Chief of Surgery at the Childrens' Hospital, Boston used to say that his anastomoses in oesophageal surgery were so good that a truck could be driven through them - a feat he used to then demónstrate with a specially sterilised children's toy truck.[276]

For those still in need of unusual facts, the head of Fallopius is still kept preserved in a bucket at the University of Turin. Should anyone think of repeating this rather unusual act of obsequies in commemorating an illustrious researcher one can only hope that the officer to whom health and safety at the place of work has been entrusted is mindful of the fact that a young researcher at the National Hospital for Nervous Disorders nearly broke her foot when she dropped a brain onto it; of course this had been deep frozen and so constituted a greater hazard than a thawed one.

PROFESSIONAL RIVALRIES

In which the authors in their examination of the subject draw attention to the points of :

(a) Pedantry

(b) Remuneration

(c) Faint Praise

(d) Adventures of a Peripatetic Professor

(e) Unsung Heroes and Cock Ups

(a) Pedantry.

The heading *otitic barotrauma* might not sound too many alarm bells these days but it was of sufficient importance to warrant a letter to be published in the British Medical Journal in 1945. The irate correspondent congratulates the author of a previous article for asserting the error of *aero-otitis media* as there is no inflammatory change. *"In the interests of accuracy and euphony the term otitic barotrauma has now taken its place and has been adopted by the R.A.F"*. Our correspondent feels obliged to draw attention to the fact that while he has no arguments about the euphony, *"otitic"* signified inflammation just as much as *"otitis"* did and that a proposal he had already made, namely *"tubo-tympanic pressure syndrome"*, should be adopted.[277] Remember, in February 1945 at the time of writing, the Second World War was still being fought.

The passage of time has not managed to sort out such problems, nor heal the acrimony which can ensue as a letter from H D Brown Kelly to the *Journal of the Royal Society of Medicine* in 1992 shows.[278] Attention is drawn to the fact that when he submitted the title to his MD thesis as being *The Diagnosis of Rhinogenic Headache* a courteous letter from the Dean informed him:

> *Rhinogenic headache means a headache productive of a nose, and I take it that your thesis holds no reference to such a phenomenon.*

We are reminded (or learn) of the fact that *genesis* is the act of producing (Gr.gennao, to produce) and "genesis" is pertaining to the generation of a thing so that terminations such as *genic* do not refer to the site of a lesion but to its production. Despite this we find throughout medical literature references to such things as *"otogenic meningitis"*, *"sinogenic headache"* and probably the most common mistake, *"bronchogenic carcinoma"*. If such an aberration presents itself at an examination viva, the reader is strongly encouraged to forcibly draw the attention of the examiner to his complete lack of understanding of the classics, quoting this chapter as a reference. The authors *guarantee* a successful outcome. It may come as a surprise, but then again it may not, to the reader that one of the authors was forced to write a strong letter to the editor of so august a journal as that of the Royal Society of Medicine pointing out an error which, had it gone uncorrected, would have done untold damage. Had there been any inaction on his part, and had this been revealed to *The Queen's English Society,* his life membership might well have revoked. Vigilance must be our watchword. For the benefit of our American readers, the letter, which was published immediately by a contrite editor, aghast at the error of his minions, is reproduced in full:

Lesions Of The Internal Auditory Meatus

I hope the authors of the article on screening for lesions of the internal auditory meatus[uu] will not consider me pedantic (![vv]*) if I remind them of the correct plural. Being fourth declension, rather than second, it is meatus, or, anglicised, meatuses. Such a publication, uncorrected, read by impressionable junior staff denied a classical education, will only serve to propage this source of irritation to radiologists.*[279]

Pedants do not necessarily confine themselves to the classics when pointing out to others the error of their ways. An anatomy professor found it *"unfortunate and discomforting"* when authors *"chose to reintroduce the term "turbinate" in place of "concha"*, citing the third edition of *Nomina Anatomica* (1966).[280] The authors' defence was that this was the term used currently by all nasal surgeons in both the U.K. and North America, with a final line: *"We hope that preclinical teachers will take note".*[281] Of course it is perfectly possible to get too clever, especially when using metaphors, as the men from the ministry found when writing their words of wisdom:

Many persons who have experienced a nuclear explosion will have diarrhoea and vomiting and should not be allowed to swamp the medical services.[282]

This is perhaps an appropriate moment to warn of the dangers of the use of the word *auriscope* as opposed to *otoscope*. As a medical student on secondment to Barnsley District General Hospital (where the Matron wore a bright red tippet and the Deputy Matron had a bow under the chin which just showed through her beard) one of your

---

uu

Robson A K, Leighton S E J, Anslow P, Milford C A. MRI as a single screening procedure for acoustic neuroma: a cost effective procedure. J Roy Soc med 1993;86:455-457.

vv

The very idea!

authors, wanting to look in his patient's ear, asked a student nurse for an auriscope. At first she looked puzzled and then her lovely face lit up and she started to rummage amongst the things on the top of the bedside locker of the old miner, finally extricating a copy of the *Daily Mirror*. Then, triumphantly opening it at the appropriate page she asked the patient his birth sign. The word *otoscope* is therefore recommended.

No work on otolaryngology would be complete without a few words on the long-standing problem of by which set of names the phenomenon of *sideropenic dysphagia* should be called - otherwise known as *"The Boring Problem of Paterson Brown Kelly and Plummer-Vinson Syndrome"*. Your authors are delighted to be in a position to at last reveal the truth, especially because, as will be seen, the true honours belong in Yorkshire. The astute reader will have realised that this is where both authors are proud to have been born. Their jingoistic fervour does not extend, however, to the extent of endorsing *Yorkshire Tea*. [ww] In fact, though well aware of the beneficial climatic effects of the so-called greenhouse effect, neither author was of the opinion that it was possible to grow tea even on the southern slopes of the southernmost hills of Yorkshire. But, of course, Yorkshire tea would probably be a lot hardier than the foreign sort. But we digress. The charitable might forgive the Americans for using the term *Plummer-Vinson Syndrome*. Plummer and Vinson were after all both colonials working at the Mayo Clinic. The fact that the disease they described had already been recorded twice before them in the United Kingdom is incidental, and can best be ascribed to youthful enthusiasm. Evidently in 1922, Vinson was Plummer's sycophantic junior who presented some work about which his boss was vaguely aware, but his ambitious nature prompted him to name it after him.[283] This was some three years after Donald Rose Paterson (an Edinburgh graduate doing missionary work in Cardiff) and Adam Brown Kelly of Glasgow both turned up to the same meeting of the Royal Society of Medicine in 1919 to describe anaemic old women with oral fissures, glosso-pharyngitis and spasm in the upper oesophagus.[284] [285] What a pity neither of them had heard about the paper written in 1913 by the eminent Bradford laryngologist, Adolf Bronner.[286] Yes, the authors who are both from Yorkshire, and one of whom (JDCB) is from Bradford, would be the first to admit that Adolf Bronner is indeed an unusual name for a Yorkshireman and would further like to bet that he kept a pretty low profile in the four years (1914-1918) subsequent to the publication of his paper.

---

ww

Tetley's *Yorkshire Tea* [R].

The Title of *Doctor* or *Mister*?

A proposal to abandon the tradition of addressing surgeons as "Mr" instead of "Dr" met with a frosty reception, it was reported in *Hospital Doctor* early in 1992.[287] The current tradition, which has never held for otolaryngologists in Edinburgh who proudly display the title *Doctor*, was defended by the Royal College of Surgeons which claimed that the custom dated back 800 years, had served the profession well, and that there was no reason for change. The controversy is nothing new, as anyone familiar with the *British Medical Journal* of Victorian times will be only too well aware. For those of our readers for whom clinical responsibilities bear too heavy to allow more than the minimum familiarity with this (and it is for those of our colleagues that this book is primarily intended) we will choose just one example, written anonymously under the title, *A Doctor, But Not M.D.* in 1876. He proclaims that *"despite of any bylaw, I shall continue to call myself doctor, for the Royal College of Physicians were trying to restrict this to holders of the degree of Doctor of Medicine"*. The worthy correspondent goes on to write that: *to attempt to confine the title of "doctor" to M.D.s of Universities is an attempt to create a medical monopoly on the part of a limited number of bodies who do not respond to all necessities of practice. If this be upheld, there can be no "doctors" made in London, the greatest medical centre in the world, except by that very exclusive and high-flying body the University of London, which reserves that title for bookworms of the highest and most exhaustive (not to say exhausted) order.*[288]

This is quite different from the position today. In fact an attacker to the 1992 article claimed that *Mister* was an inverted form of snobbery, singling out the highly qualified doctor from his peers. In more recent times (historically speaking) it has been the custom to restrict the use of this title to those who have passed their Fellowship examination. The librarian of the Royal College of Surgeons was even quoted in the *Hospital Doctor* article as saying that *"he would be rather sad to see "Mr" go because it doesn't harm anyone and these nice little idiosyncrasies in a sense make life worthwhile"*. Your authors do not have such strong feelings as to consider that the worthwhileness of life depends on the subject, despite the flurry of correspondence which flooded the medical journals. One penned a reply but forgot to post it. The other held that were dentists to start using calling themselves *doctor* - an argument that was running parallel, then the title would be so devalued that everybody might as well be Dr - or Mr. This didn't do him any good as his brother, a dentist, simply stopped lending him his sportscar.

The late, great Kenneth Harrison once asked a disciple *"Why do you think I always use a post-aural incision rather than an endaural one?"* A flood of answers ensued:

> *Because it is better cosmetically and follows Langer's lines,*
> *Because it never gives a fistula,*
> *It is easier to stitch up,*
> *It doesn't cause neuralgia,*
> *There is less tension in the wound,*
> *There is less post-operative pain"*

All these answers were met with a dismissive negative. When at last the registrars gave up and asked for the real reason, the Master smiled and slowly replied:

> *Well, I suppose really it's because I've always used it.*

(b) Remuneration.

Fees have always been a thorny subject, not least when one considers what professionals in other fields might be making in considerably less time (though with perhaps more effort). We are told the story of a Lancashire man who consulted a colleague privately after going with a prostitute and who was worried he might have caught something. He sought the opinion of an Ear, Nose & Throat surgeon because that is where the action had taken place. After the requisite tests he was assured that he need have no worries, but as he had been seen privately there would be a bill to pay. Taking pity on the man, the kindly and benevolent otolaryngologist charged him his minimum rate, to be met with a gasp of disbelief. His fears that even this was beyond his pocket were put to rest when the man cheerfully announced that it was cheaper than the prostitute. One has not only to compare the fees which might be obtainable in the practice of otolaryngology with other professions, but also in looking over a period of time, with other costs. For example in 1902 an Urban Council unanimously passed a resolution that:

> *In cases notified as diphtheria in which swabbings taken by the medical attendant*
> *are confirmed by the bacteriologist to the Council a fee of 10s 6d shall be paid*
> *to the medical attendant.*[289]

To put this in some sort of historical context this was a third to a half of many a worker's weekly wage. However, in comparison to this, the announcement, admittedly thirty years before from the Committee of Westminster Hospital that registrars

> *who have hitherto done the duties of these appointments gratuitously will be remunerated; the sum of eighty pounds has accordingly been voted for the purpose, but only for the ensuing year.*[290]

Tony Bull and Ian Mackay are the two smoothy London surgeons who run the excellent Rhinoplasty course at Gray's Inn Road every year. Rhinoplasty, of course, is a bit of a money spinner,[xx] and expertise in the art can almost be *"the potentiality of growing rich beyond the dreams of avarice.*[yy] Ian tells a lovely story about Tony Bull when he was about to go on one of his many continental trips and decided to apply for an American Express *Gold Card*. Evidently the agent was a young girl who was unaware that Tony was a wealthy Harley Street surgeon, and told him that before anyone could be given a gold card they must answer a few personal questions. He said that he quite understood and so she started to ask him about his income, starting rather tentatively at wondering whether he earned in excess of £20,000.

"Oh yes", he replied without hesitation.

"Well then", she said with a little less diffidence, *"Do you earn more than £50,000?"*

"Yes", he replied.

Feeling more confident now she ventured: *"Alright then Sir, would you say that you made more than £100,000?"*

At this point Mr Bull hesitated and there was a pregnant silence, broken eventually by him admitting that it was rather difficult to say; some weeks he did, some weeks he didn't.

[xx]

Rhino, as any reader of Billy Bunter will know, is an old term for money and many allege that it is from this that the term rhinoplasty derives.

[yy]

This is a quote from our lexicographer pal, Dr Johnson, on the occasion of the sale of Thrales' brewery in 1781. Samuel Johnson's girlfriend was Mrs Thrale and the good doctor was made chief executor. Boswell tells us:

> On being asked what he really considered to be the value of the property which was to be disposed of answered:
>> *Sir, we are not here to sell a parcel of vats and boilers, but the potentiality of growing rich beyond the dreams of avarice.*

Time was to prove him true: Thrales became Courage Brewery!

When considering the vexed question of filthy lucre, one should obviously bear in mind that there has always been a contrast between the high earnings of those at the top of the profession and those struggling their way up. Medicine differs in this in no way from the other professions where the bright young newcomer has to serve his time before reaching the remuneration of the seasoned campaigner. The profession of prostitution may well prove an exception, though the authors would not like to be too definite upon this, their application for a research grant having been turned down[zz]. What has changed nowadays is that formerly the difference between a well-established practitioner and his apprentice was in the cut and quality of clothes rather than the mode of dress and both were for the most part distinguishable from those they treated. Today neither is the case. Someone walking the wards in pre-War days would notice stiff erect formal figures soberly dressed (the doctors)[aaa] surrounded by bent, broken Lowry-like characters clutching dressings to various parts and oozing blood, pus etc (the patients). How different the scene is today! A bronzed, permed young Adonis bounds into the Sports Medicine Clinic and after being counselled by a variety of *health care professionals*[bbb] (and no doubt receiving a few free condoms) asks the doctor for some embrocation (no doubt using a fancy word learnt at the health club) and a support bandage for his "sports injury". The doctor, after a sleepless night in an uncleaned on-call room bereft of bed linen stares blankly ahead, a sheaf of job applications spilling out of a tattered white coat which, in the way that plumbers and electricians strap their tools onto belts, serves as a scaffolding for a panoply of medical instruments, trousers crumpled and unshaven. Some of the men are even worse.

Of course when speaking of remuneration one must consider the non-pecuniary

---

[zz]

One of the authors did receive two grants some time ago to research prostitution in Portugal. He learnt a lot, and the benefits of his toil may be read: Young J R. *Prostitution In Portugal*. Br Med Stud J 1969;2:19.

[aaa]

The readers who suspend belief should take a look at some old Residents photographs.

[bbb]

The mother of one of the authors has a very dim view of all forms of counselling, having lived through the hazards of being bombed, though not evacuated, during the War. She points out there was no "counselling" then, and it didn't *seem* to do anybody any harm. The authors agree, but must point out that were it to be abolished, the counsellors might well suffer - would they be harmed by not being counselled then?

rewards as well. Delightful unwitting testimony to the subtle use of influence to procure additional benefit is given by Sir Frederick Mott when relating the practice of a colleague, Sir William Broadbent. Describing him as *"that great and experienced physician"*, he relates how he had noticed that frequently in the houses of the wealthy it was difficult to obtain suitable food for patients, owing, he held to the failure of the chefs to understand, and the lack of authority of the nurse. He would, therefore, knowing the great importance attached to proper food being given to his patient, go into the kitchen and instruct the cook in the preparation of suitable food. Afterwards he would, when visiting, *"ask for the food to be brought that he might taste it"*.[291] Neither author has adopted this for use in domiciliary visits, but would be interested to hear from any reader who can vouch for its efficacy.

Frank Stansfield of the anatomy cramming course fame, used to hold that the only function of Waldeyer's ring was to provide custard-coloured Rolls-Royces for ENT surgeons. In this he was probably not strictly correct. A well-known Australian surgeon called his Rolls-Royce *Grommets* - because they had paid for it. Tonsillectomy might, in the view of some, fulfil a similar function. Whilst demonstrating a new instrument he had devised for tonsillectomy, Mr J F O'Malley told the audience that he was in the habit of operating on thirty cases in the morning at his hospital in two hours.[292] Not all ENT surgeons are so conventional in their tastes and there is none better to illustrate this than Sir William Milligan (for even the eccentric Draffin possessed a couple of Rolls-Royces). The department in Manchester where he worked still treasures the picture of him directing the traffic in the centre of Manchester, and local children used to wait after school for him to pass by to laugh at him.[293] One should be aware of the dangers of appearing too unconventional - in the words Alan Bennett puts into the mouth of a character seeing the doctor who is about to manage her case:

> *He had one of those zip-up cardigans, which didn't inspire confidence.*[294]

It has been customary for eminent surgeons to advertise their eminence and adroitness at the operating table by inviting colleagues (usually for a fee) to watch them operating. The dress of such spectators should be, it is advised by Shambaugh in his famous textbook, trussed like a mummy with the arms completely immobilised by the sides rather like a straight-jacket.[295] This was presumably to prevent the surgical equivalent of a "back seat driver". It may in earlier times have also served to protect the innocent bystander for it is reported that with a single cut, one of the nineteenth century's greatest surgeons not only amputated the patient's leg as intended but also managed to remove three fingers of the assistant and his own coat-tail.[296] A case has also been reported where the surgeon cut so vigorously that he managed to perform inadvertent self-circumcision! Jacques Joseph took the practice a stage further when he dismissed his spectators during crucial parts of the operation so that they would not learn his "trade secrets". The authors are as yet unaware as to whether his operating theatre nurses ever divulged this information and for what price. Cottle was so irritated at having to be one of an audience of twenty or so spectators for one of Joseph's nasal operations that in desperation to obtain a good view he bought all twenty seats. Two seats at a fancy restaurant with the nurse might have yielded better results. Such behaviour has not been confined to the operating theatre. Thomas Braidwood who opened the first school for the deaf in this country kept his teaching methods a family secret although they were published after his death by his son as *Instruction of the Deaf and Dumb* (1809).[297] Of course, sometimes education and the dissemination of information can have results which might not be received in the manner in which they were intended. The great Lord Baden-Powell wrote warning of:

> the "rutting season", when young men are attracted to women. This disagreeable phase troubles some fellows to an alarming amount of depression or excitement which often lasts for several months.[298]

Well nobody should have any difficulty with getting to grips with that, but later on he comes onto much shakier ground when he (as a completely non-medical person, remember) draws the analogy with measles:

> Indeed in occasional cases it goes on for a few years. I get lots of letters from young fellows who have never been told what to expect when they are growing into manhood..... I have been able to reassure them and help them to take it calmly and to get over it just as they would get over the measles.

(c) Faint Praise.

> To those who, like us, are apt to go a bit too far.
> Which, as we know, is usually just far enough.

Of course your authors would be the first to acknowledge that not all forms of condemnation are meant with malice aforethought. Witness the remark made by Capital Radio to the effect that Madonna, after being struck on the head by her husband Sean

Penn, was rushed to hospital for a brain scan *but nothing was found*. It is not always said unwittingly: Randolph Churchill once had to go ito hospital for the investigation of a tumour, which was subsequently pronounced not malignant. Evelyn Waugh remarked how brilliant it had been of medical science *"to find the one part of Randolph that is not malignant"*.

J F O'Malley proudly introduced in 1912 his new instrument to the section of laryngology of the Royal Society of Medicine. It was a new type of tonsillectomy guillotine, which he named his *tonsillotome*, and he assured the assembled audience that during the past year he had used it on almost a thousand cases with very beneficial results. In the ensuing discussion Dr Watson-Williams provided what might have been predicted by the shrewd or cynical, namely that he:

> *was sure that the principle of the instrument was the right one; more than a year ago he had designed a similar instrument, and more recently Professor Ballenger had shown him his original tonsil forceps, which was very much like his own design.*[299]

In this he was only confirming the theory subsequently neatly formulated by J Stokes of University College Hospital that the time taken for a new idea to gain acceptance can be divided, like the ages of man, into seven phases:

1. I don't believe it
2. It won't work
3. The numbers are not statistically significant
4. It's dangerous
5. It's not possible to make it generally available
6. Of course, we've known it all the time
7. Actually we thought of it first ourselves.

The above phenomenon is more likely to occur where events are widespread not only in time but also geographically. Cramped together in a metropolis such as London, it would be less easy to miss something new - or, as Sir St Clair Thomson put it: *"But in London, where we have such good opportunities of becoming conscious of one another's imperfections..."*.[300]

These imperfection may take many forms. Lennox Browne (1841-1902) was not put on the staff of the Throat Hospital, Golden Square owing, it was considered, to his reputation of being somewhat unscrupulous. His obituary makes interesting reading:

> *He contributed to the literature of his subject with considerable frequency, and,
> it need hardly be said, was always ready to join in the controversies of the day...
> He was possessed of a keen intellect and great technical acumen, with a masterful
> force of character which helped him over many obstacles. It must be admitted
> that he was essentially combative and intolerant of opposition, and was apt to
> fall back upon his exceptional dialectic power rather than on that conciliatory
> tact which his remarkable personality would have made so powerful.*[301]

One can only wonder just what was actually meant, especially by "masterful force of character" One is reminded of the conjugation of the reflexive verb "to be firm" which goes:

> I am firm
> You are stubborn
> He is pig-headed

Even the great Sir Charles Sherrington could not resist a slight dig when he came to write of his friend and colleague Sir Charles Ballance, stating: *"If as he grew older he seemed a little liable to "preach" somewhat.*[302] One wonders what he really wanted to say! The same might be said of the description of Arthur Cheatle (1867-1929) as having *"a charming personality with occasional inflexible opinions".*[303]

To those who know Bill Gill, the following may not sound so terrible, especially to those who have had experience of massive Outpatient clinics, but to the bleeding heart "counsellors" it probably does. Bill was, in the presence of one of the authors, being consulted by a Lancashire couple about their child. The mother said that her child had a nose bleed, and, after examining him, Bill confirmed that the problem was amenable to surgery and that he would wash out his sinuses, remove his tonsils and adenoids, and at the same time cauterise his nose. There followed a lengthy discussion during the course of which he repeated what his advice was. The mother was clearly not impressed and began to remonstrate before being bustled out of the room by her husband. Bill turned to the author and said:

> *John, it's a wonder some of these people don't bring a picnic hamper!*

When a similar situation arose, the consultant with whom one of the authors was working had the devastating reply to being questioned whether it would be possible to explain some medical condition:

Of course, do you have seven years to spare?

Criticism has not always been so subtle, as is revealed by the remarks made by the *Edinburgh Medical and Surgical Journal* on the appearance of Volume 4 of *Transactions*, a rival journal, being that of the Royal College of Physicians[ccc]:

> *The College now and then finds a little leisure, and now and then feels a little zeal, for the cultivation of medical science. These paroxsyms of exertion occur, it is true, but seldom and at distant periods, like the visits of influenza, and their exciting causes are not always discernible by the multitude. 250 years had passed away....when the first fit came on and the first volume of its Transactions was published in 1768....and now after the silent lapse of 28 years more, the 4th volume comes forth....[It is] not as good as Medical Essays of Edinburgh or Medical Observations and Inquiries of London.... The inferior merit of the present volume will not admit of dispute....*[304]

The obituary of Sir Henry Trentham Butlin, Bart (1843-1912) in the *British Medical Journal* runs to over five pages, including a full page photograph.[305] A description of his achievements, which are indeed notable, for he was President of the Royal College of Surgeons of England in 1909 and re-elected twice, is followed by eulogies from five of his colleagues. If only he had named an instrument he might be better known today or at least have had some more tangible form of memorial in the fashion of the general surgeon whose obituary follows his. It was recorded that this chap's work for the Chester Infirmary was publicly acknowledged by a presentation taking the form of *a valuable antique clock and candelabra, a beautiful silver tea and coffee service and a cheque for £200.*[306] This was quite a lot of money, for in 1912 the *Lancet* was carrying advertisements for assistant surgeons with an *annual* remuneration of £80. Nevertheless, Sir Henry was not, it seems, shy in sounding his own trumpet and having an eye to the main chance. He

---

[ccc]

Founded in 1518, the College produced only six volumes of *Transactions* between 1768 and 1820. In contrast, the house journal of the Royal Society of Medicine, established in 1809, was always a prestigious journal and probably the only one in the early 19th century which refereed papers submitted for publication.

began a lecture delivered at St Bartholomew's Hospital, 20 November 1901, with the words:

> *Gentlemen, I have for some time past had it in my mind to lecture on the removal of the ovaries for malignant disease of the breast.*[307]

Close examination of his presentation reveals however that the main case which he describes was thought by many of his colleagues as *"a proper case on which to try the experiment"* and it transpires that in fact he has little or no experience of the subject at all, admitting that .... *"generally speaking, we agreed that the operation should be practised in that case. My colleague, Mr Lockwood, removed the ovaries and tubes".*

Professional rivalries frequently surface and, in the authors' opinion, exchanges at public meetings cannot be bettered for the one-upmanship which such encounters engender. Dan McKenzie had the idea of inserting soft metal tubes into the nose immediately after nasal surgery with the aim of avoiding the blockage which was caused by the postoperative packing.[308] At the subsequent discussion following their presentation at the Royal Society of Medicine, Mr Harmer said that he had been using rubber tubes in the nose for four years; Dr Jobson Horne said he was glad these tubes were being *re-introduced*!

Pop Hastings was praised for his ability to almost complete a mastoidectomy with three strokes of his gouge. He admitted that he had the largest number of facial palsies but considered that this was *more than offset by the fact that his cavities were also the cleanest*. Of course something like that could never happen nowadays, as we are all supplied so well with modern electric drills. The reader should note that although such drills *are* made by the Zimmer company, this firm *do not* make zimmer frames. No doubt as a result of many pointless enquiries, they have resorted to producing a pamphlet explaining that they, the Zimmer company, *do not* make Zimmer walking frames, which are made by another company, *not* called Zimmer.

(d) Adventures of a Peripatetic Professor (With Advice to Missionaries of Otolaryngology.

We are indebted to Professor Sir Donald F N Harrison, who has covered virtually every aspect of the globe during the time he was Professor of Otolaryngology at the Royal National Throat, Nose and Ear Hospital (and hence for a period the sole professor of our subject in this country) for contributing this section. It seems more appropriate to record the contribution of our country's greatest living exponent of ENT and perhaps one of its best known ambassadors in something more than a footnote and for this contribution the authors join with the reader in thanking him most heartily. It was brought home to us both how true the saying is that medical eminence is not always solely the consequence of chance and fortuitous circumstance (though the reader's impression from some of the contents of this chapter especially might well give that impression) but also the result of dedication, drive and perseverance. Your authors should perhaps not have been surprised to be receiving messages by fax and telephone exhorting them to greater effort; how many editors one wonders are in the position of receiving "camera-ready copy" [ddd] by return of post?

Practical Tips from Sir Donald:

1. Eat and drink sparingly, for air-induced hangovers are not to be recommended prior to three weeks of intensive lecturing. On the other hand, when on the ground, alcohol may be needed to maintain that "bright approach" which is an integral element of we benevolent Britishers - in my own case this can be maintained for about three days at a time. I have never been a great or imaginative eater and have always lost weight when away on trips. This has been frequently associated with constipation, which may be regarded by many afflicted with the opposite problem as a boon. There was one time, however, when under the influence of alcohol I did eat some oysters in Bangkok which produced a nasty attack of cholera. It is no fun lecturing three or four times a day with permanent tenesmus. I do take the precaution of always carrying a DIY toilet repair kit which, as all the older cisterns were made in Sheffield, serves to keep the water running in a variety of international settings.

2. Just as my DIY toilet kit never leaves my possession, neither do my slides. If you had had the experience of your slide case containing two hundred precious illustrations for an imminent lecture springing open whilst strolling around a swimming pool in Jamaica (and there can be few of us who have not experienced this at some time or another) then you would do the same.

---

ddd

Whatever that might be - here for once our American readers may well have the advantage. Much good may it do them.

3. Whilst being sparing with the food and drink, do, however, collect as many travelling socks and any other gifts you can, for although pretty useless in the air, they are very much sought after at car boot sales where my younger daughter succeeded in disposing of my entire collection numbering more than one hundred in about ten minutes.

4. If you have been lucky enough to have your fare paid for by an airline there is an understandable feeling of professional responsibility which, except in the most urgent situation, should be suppressed. I had been persuaded in 1977 to give the opening address at the World Congress in Otolaryngology. This was held in Buenos Aires and I was provided with a first class air ticket on Air Argentina. This flew from London via Barcelona and Rio. The cabin crew followed the usual formula found on South American airlines of pouring several strong drinks into the passengers and then departing from view whilst they held their own party. All was well until we had left Spain and were several hours over the Atlantic when, first in Spanish and then in desperate English, came a call for a doctor. I had already had several experiences of the hazards inherent in admitting to being a member of the medical profession, let alone a professor, but unwisely I revealed my identity and immediately was hustled behind the curtain separating the first class compartment from the seething masses crammed into the standard section. An attractive young lady lay groaning on one of the front seats. Using the clearly unconcerned male steward as an interpreter I elicited the fact that she was complaining of abdominal pain. Thinking that it may be an ectopic pregnancy (I had always wanted to be a gynaecologist, but there were more openings in ENT) I tried to find whether she might be pregnant - this immediately silenced the milling throng of passengers behind me, but she remained uncommunicative. This left me somewhat in a quandary, so, drawing on my recollections of television doctor programmes I exclaimed in a loud voice my sorrow at not being able to give her anything for her pain as I did not have my black bag with me. This seemed to convey the right note of caring. Without further prompting the steward produced a couple of syringes like a magician with rabbits out of a hat, proclaiming that injections were always carried. Aeroplane lighting leaves much to be desired, but there was little point in trying to read the small print on the syringes as it was all in Spanish. Expectations were high, so, after anointing her buttocks with whisky, I gave her the first injection. She quickly fell into a deep sleep, following which her friend joined the crew behind the curtain. Three hours later at the request of the crew, and,

supposedly, the patient, in went the second injection. At Rio I was asked by the captain to remain on board whilst the airport doctor made his diagnosis. He was also non plussed but left me with a further two ampoules to be injected before we arrived in Argentina. On disembarkation there I was met by my host, the president of the congress, but interrupted by the attractive young lady who thanked me for the injections and gave me her telephone number imploring me to telephone her so that she could thank me properly. I never did succeed in explaining to my hosts what might, on reflection, seem to be an implausible story, nor how she so quickly managed to acquire a knowledge of English.

(What Sir Donald has studiously avoided mentioning is practical advice to our readers regarding sexual encounters in areas of high risk such as Thailand, Malaysia etc. We are of course referring to the phenomenon of heat exhaustion which can occur under conditions of extreme physical effort with concurrent deprivation of fluid. One of your authors learned of a method of avoiding this danger whilst still enjoying the pleasures of the flesh whilst serving in the Middle East. It is of such cunning that it is thought that the origins derive from the Teutonic Knights and the days of the Crusades. The male member is thrust from a kneeling position into the right armpit of a woman[eee]. She is seated in front of him, and proceeds to shuffle a pack of cards. Both parties fortify themselves with copious volumes of gin and tonic from a jug placed to their left. This may be recommended as a useful form of SAFE SEX - but like all, it is only really safe so long as you don't get caught[fff]. But we digress, and return you to Sir Donald.)

5.   Assurances that all the equipment you could possible need is available must be treated with caution, unless you are in a military hospital. A lateral rhinotomy in Kutching, Sarawak was timed at six minute bursts since that was the life span of the headlight torch batteries when working at full power. I have known anaesthetists sleep with their endotracheal tubes, such has their scarcity been

---

[eee]

Our American readers should note that it is regarded as a point of etiquette to seek the prior consent of the lady in question.

[fff]

It is also important should one lose control or balance to fall over to the right or the jug might be knocked over.

(one of your authors once knew an anaesthetist who slept with his *Resusci-Anne*, but it was not thought that this was because it was in such short supply that it was in danger of being stolen).

In conclusion, as an ambassador for academic ENT-Head & Neck Surgery, I consider myself extremely fortunate to have travelled so widely at a time when our specialty was developing and few surgeons were prepared to venture into relatively primitive situations. The ability to meet and sometimes select enthusiastic young people to return with me to the United Kingdom for training made these visits really worthwhile. It not only raised standards but helped to end the practice of visiting operators who suffered from the drawback that when all went well, then the procedure appeared easy; if it went badly, then reputations were lost. The hospitality and enthusiasm shown by locals on my trips remains one of the highlights of my professional life, and my wife and I often comment that we have more good friends abroad than at home.

Professor Sir Donald Harrison PhD MD FRCS

(e) Unsung Heroes and Cock Ups.

Benjamin Babington discovered hereditary haemorrhagic telangiectasia in 1865, (refresh your memory by rereading page 95) some thirty years before Rendu in 1896 and well before Osler in 1901. As it is also considered that he developed the first laryngoscope, many years before Garcia, he must be a strong contender along with Draffin as being one of the unluckiest ENT pioneers.[309] As amply demonstrated by Draffin, an invention does not necessarily lead to wealth and professional advancement, and this was certainly the experience of J H Curtis (1778-1860). It is accepted that he was somewhat extravagant in his claims for his acoustical chair but nevertheless he attracted a powerful clientele. Unfortunately for him he was attacked by Wilde and some of the more orthodox practitioners and died in penury.[310] He was thus denied the opportunity of the immortality obtained by those wealthy enough to leave legacies to perpetuate their name. An example is Herbert Tilley, who bequeathed £800 to the Royal Ear Hospital for the appropriately named Herbert Tilley museum.[311] There are other ways of letting people know just who you are. Sir Felix Semon was favoured with royal patronage, something which he wanted to be certain would not be lost on newcomers to the subject of otolaryngology. Consequently, he printed a picture of himself and the king on a hunting expedition in the textbook he wrote. It is not always plain sailing, though. It is recorded that Duncan Gibb's assumption of the title of Baronet was *"the source of much annoyance and trouble to him and, no doubt, it injured his professional advancement, while the investigation connected with it occupied much of his time".*[312]

Before the development of "pull-ups" or pedicled colon grafts for oesophageal replacement a Texan[ggg] surgeon suggested that a tube of skin from the penis turned inside out should be used. This, he claimed, was because of its distensibility and unique ability to stretch to the required dimensions when in situ. The plan was then to bury the flayed lingam under the skin of the lower abdominal wall in a sort of tunnel. No mention was made of prophylactic bromide, it having been assumed that the usual age groups at which oesophageal cancer occurs would preclude the proband from worrying (which goes to show that elderly Texans have different priorities to elderly Yorkshiremen!). On reflection, few men would have too much cause to worry with their penis constantly buried in a tunnel of abdominal skin - even if it were their own. This in turn reminds one of the authors of the written FRCS examination paper he sat in 1975 in which the first question was *Describe syphilis of the ear*. He began penning the line:

There was an old man from Nantucket

but then thought better of it and put a line through the sentence. Two days later in Liverpool, he met the examiner who said that it was still discernible through the crossing out and it had given him the only laugh he had had whilst marking the papers. Nonetheless your author failed[hhh].

Dr C.L. Joiner[iii] reminds us that one of the complications of Hereditary Haemorrhagic Telangiectasia consequent to the continued loss of blood used to be iron

---

[ggg]

Texas is the U.S.A's equivalent of Yorkshire.

[hhh]

So much for the anonymity of the FRCS question papers. How did the examiner know 147 = JRY? Green ink.

[iii]

Contemporary

deficiency anaemia. In the past this was described as *chlorosis* (the green sickness) as it tended to occur in the poor who suffered not only from anaemia but also lack of sunlight and malnutrition. Pathologists of the time unhesitatingly attributed it to compression of the liver from tight corsetry and managed to describe a characteristic groove over the chondral surface of the liver caused by this.[313] Whilst we are on the subject of haematology we should perhaps relate the case told to us by Dr Paul L F Giangrande[iii] of a man who was referred to him shortly after he was appointed to a consultancy in Oxford. Paul, who is an extraordinary clever fellow as any who were in his year at medical school will testify, had little difficulty in utilising a variety of erudite tests and investigations to make the diagnosis of leukaemia. He was, however, concerned that the man had delayed so long before seeking medical advice and confessed to being a little surprised that someone should wait for so long after developing lumps in the axillae, for there is normally a high ambient intelligence quotient in Oxford. The answer was quite simple. The man had taken up golf and thought the lumps were muscles developing. One of the authors can have sympathy with this misconception for following a prolonged period of cross country skiing he developed a large swelling around the abdomen which despite complete abstinence from skiing or any form of severe physical exercise persists.

A man's ear which was bitten off after a pub fight was kept in the fridge of the local police station, it was reported in a national newspaper. The faithful Messrs Plod were *"waiting for the owner to appear and allow surgeons to sew it back on"*.[314]

[iii]

Contemporary,

THE "FRINGES" OF OUR SUBJECT, INCLUDING THE ROLE OF INVALID COOKERY

In which the authors draw attention to some of the more interesting forms of "fringe medicine" which have been used in the past AND provide a valuable list of invalid recipes, document the value of adequate nutrition in the care of the sick &c &c.

(a) Homeopathy and Herbalism.

It is not without some poignancy that the authors embark on a chapter considering the phenomenon of homeopathy, stricken as they are by the loss through nervous collapse, exhaustion and bankruptcy of their friend and colleague Herbert Arkwright. He was one of the few, and possible the last, homeopathic orthopaedic specialists. His minuscule plaster of Paris casts were to be often seen around city streets the length and breadth of West Yorkshire. Miners, woolspinners, railwaymen - they all brought their broken bones for him to heal but, dogged by ill health and bad luck, he finally succumbed. In this his misfortune was only surpassed by his half cousin, the famous blues singer Whistlin' Willy Arkright who failed to find salvation at the hands of either conventional or homeopathic urologists.

The medicinal value of plants &c is well-known. What is perhaps less well-known (except, it is hoped to the natives of Tahiti) is that the flower of *Hibiscus brackenridgei*, when worn over the right ear, signifies there that one is looking for a mate. Widespread knowledge of things like that could make computer dating agencies bankrupt. The Rangoon Creeper contains quisqualic acid, which is used to treat intestinal parasites. In contrast, skin rashes can be treated with *Hibiscus* petals (but only from the darker flowered forms of course). Should there be any risk of confusion, the reader is exhorted to make use of the S. American ginger plant which is used in various ways by indigenous peoples to treat fever, coughs, sores and wounds, inflammations, intestinal worms *and* snake bites. This plant would probably come a close-second, or even beat the Lipstick tree at all-round usefulness competitions. The latter is of more interest to our specialty in that it not only has antiseptic and antivenereal properties, but the leaves can be used on cuts to help reduce scarring. When used as a gargle, it is effective on tonsillitis.

(b) Invalid Cookery.

With the crowding of the medical curriculum in recent years with items whose value is not easily apparent to your authors, (who, finding themselves confronted in a situation where further medical help was not readily available would, they have to admit, probably not be the best medical men to counsel a victim of AIDS[kkk]) the time spent on the study of the invalid diet has been sadly neglected. It is the aim of this chapter to redress this balance, and, in so doing, not only illuminate some of the darker corners of this subject hitherto neglected for some of our readers but also provide some useful tips for their wives.

In so doing, they readily admit not to being the first in this field, for the great and good Sir Frederick Mott, lecturer on Morbid Psychology at the University of Birmingham was writing in 1936 of the influence of food and its presentation on health. He reminded the reader of *Cookery Illustrated and Household Management* how a savoury odour of cooked food effects through the sense of smell a psychic process, which, starting the desire to eat, causes a flow of the digestive juices but *"if the odour of the food is unsavoury , or the food has neither flavour nor savour, and there is little or no desire to eat, this appetite juice does not flow"*.[315] He further elaborates in a style which might well not be found inappropriate in a modern ladies' magazine such as *Cosmopolitan* and which underlies the lie that medical men in former years paid no, or little attention to the psychological aspects of illness[lll]. We can do no better than quote his words verbatim:

> *The sense of sight also plays an important part in the psychological anticipation stage of eating a meal. The food should not only please the sense of smell, but also the sense of sight, by the way it is put on the table; the clean table cloth, the napkin, the hot plates, and the garnishing of the dish with parsley, watercress etc all help to promote a pleasant psychic state and the flow of appetite juices, whereas a slovenly and dirty or unpleasing table promotes a feeling of disgust and a failure of the flow of the appetite juices. An unvitiated palate is Nature's best guide for the nutrition of the individual.....a pleasant gastronomic surprise by a wife to a tired and irritable husband on coming home will often be an appetising tonic, and sometimes even be the means of preventing domestic quarrels.*

It is unfortunate that publishing difficulties preclude the authors being able to present the above advice to the reader on one of those small magnets so often found in the shape

---

[kkk]

A disease of American origin recently imported into Great Britain subsequent to the time spent by the authors as medical undergraduates.

[lll]

Despite the lack of formal courses on "counselling" in the medical curriculum!

of a number or small animal which are used to stick to the door of the domestic refrigerator. We suggest instead that the reader take scissors and paste to his spare copy of this volume and effect the same result. The very diligent may like to stick a transparent adhesive tape such as *Sellotape*[mmm] over the finished product to achieve what we are led to believe is a *Wash 'n' Wipe* surface.

> Learning Point
> There are two chief points to remember when preparing the invalid's diet: food is part of the cure and so must be made nourishing and digestible, containing those elements demanded by the patient's condition; in sickness one has little appetite, and must be tempted by dainty dishes, delicately made and attractively served.

We make the following available to our readership but trust to the sense of fair play we know to be inherent in all not to utilise a photocopier machine to the detriment of further sales of this volume.

Light Meals

Unsweetened calves' foot jelly, served on an ice cream plate, with a slice of lemon and thin wheaten wafers or buttered rusks.

Clear mutton broth with custard dice, served in a bouillon cup accompanied by fingers of brown toast.

Lamb mousse, cold, with lettuce hearts and buttered crispbread.

More Substantial Meals

Calves' Sweetbreads (baked)
Ingredients: Sweetbreads, egg and breadcrumbs, or flour; fat bacon; salted water.
Method: Put the sweetbreads in warm salted water for half an hour, take them out and

---

mmm

Our Australian readers amusingly call this *Durex*, a custom we consider to be not without its dangers.

drop them into fast-boiling salted water for 2 minutes. Take them out and dry well. Dip them in egg and bread-crumbs or flour. Place them in a pan with a little butter on top, cover with greased paper, and bake in a slow oven for 30 minutes or so, according to size.

Sheep's Head, Boiled
Ingredients: 1 sheep's head, 2 oz butter, 2 oz flour, half pint milk, half pint stock, pepper and salt, 2 tablespoonfuls chopped parsley, 1 teaspoonful powdered sage.

Method: Remove all the soft bones near the nostrils of head, also take out the brain. Put the head and brain into a very large bowl of cold water and salt, and if possible leave to stand overnight, if not, for 2 hours, then wash the head thoroughly well in cold water. Put into a large pan, cover with cold water and allow to boil; cook slowly for two and a half to three hours. The brain can be put in about 1 hour before head is cooked. Take head out and cut all meat from the bones, skin the tongue and put all on to a hot dish, keep warm. Chop brain and parsley, melt margarine in pan, add flour and cook for a minute, add milk and stock (from cooking head). Stir till boiling, add pepper, salt, brain, sage and parsley and put carefully over meat on dish. If not wishing to serve head hot, the meat can be chopped, pepper, salt, sage and a little butter added, and put into meat pots.

Invalid Drinks

Albumen Water
Ingredients: three quarters cupful boiled and chilled water; the white of an egg; 1 teaspoonful lemon juice; one and a quarter teaspoonfuls sugar.

Method: Combine the ingredients in a glass jar, shake thoroughly until well mixed, then strain, and serve cold. If permitted, a few grains of salt may be added.

Prune Water
Ingredients: half pound prunes; 1 lemon; water and sugar.

Method: Soak the prunes in cold water overnight, place them in a jar with the rind of the lemon and steam until tender, strain and press or squeeze out the juice of the prunes, sweeten to taste, and add the strained juice of the lemon.

Beef Tea
Ingredients: 1lb buttock steak, 1 pint cold water, pinch salt.

Method: Scrape the steak, put into a jar with the water and salt, allow to stand covered over for half an hour, stir frequently, cover with a greased paper, and steam for three or four hours. Strain through a coarse strainer and serve with a few breadcrumbs or fingers of toast if the patient can take these.

EDUCATION AND TRAINING

In which the authors not only document the failures of the past but reveal the answers for the future to the problems besetting our specialty.
AND
The paradox of "Publish and be Praised"
AND
The Role of the Moustache in Otolaryngology

(in REVERSE order!)

137

(a) The Role of the Moustache in Otolaryngology.

In this, we are authors attempting to remedy the neglect of this subject which has sadly been a feature of many textbooks, even of some which have achieved a degree of success and reputation. Of course, during the First World War it was compulsory to wear a moustache - until a famous actor refused, fearing it would permanently damage not only his reputation but also his upper lip. However, whilst researching deep in the stacks of the library of the Royal Society of Medicine looking out photographs of the great and the good (which are not necessarily the same, as those who have reached this far in the book will realise!) and correlating moustache-length with reputation, we thought that by so doing, we were depriving somebody of material for an MD degree! Well, it cannot be much less use than trawling through somebody else's series of acoustics trying to find some common thread. So, we said we would leave it for another time/person/edition.

(b) The Life without Examination is not worth Living.

Plato said this, but then he did not have to memorise the relations of the lesser sac or write short notes on the carpal tunnel like budding otolaryngologists who want the diploma of *Fellowship of the Royal College of Surgeons*. Of course, examinations and the diplomas consequent upon them can be given more importance than is warranted. Nowhere was this more aptly illustrated than in the case of the young man who was seeking the services of a prostitute. On learning the price he complained that it was too much. The girl was quite affronted as she was, she claimed, an MRCP - a Member of the Royal College of Prostitutes. With a certain amount of disdain she advised him to go further along the street where he might find something more within his price range. He did this, and on finding a cheaper girl, questioned whether the price was lower because she was not an MRCP. She agreed that this was the case but pointed out that she had only failed on the oral.

The special qualities required by an otolaryngologist are not easily defined and even more difficult to quantify. Current leaders of the profession can take consolation from the fact that their illustrious forebears wrestled long and hard with this problem, sometimes (but not very often, for many of these men on being given strong drugs, would hallucinate vividly in grey) coming up with sensationally revolutionary ideas (for the time). More often the consensus has seemed to be that an aspiring otolaryngologist should model himself on his chief in the time honoured tradition of the apprentice, a system on which both the Royal College of Surgeons and the Worshipful Society of Apothecaries were based. If he showed the right qualities, by which of course are meant the qualities shown by oneself, then one's protegée might, with the right encouragement and backing achieve success and take his place with his former masters. But he probably would not achieve quite the same level of eminence or respect - for the new generation never work quite as hard as the old, who never had it so easy as the young.

It was not the intention in writing this piece to recount the deeds of the famous, but in the case of Wm Johnson Walsham (1847-1903), an exception will be made, as it illustrates some of the differences in practice over the years within our specialty. He began as an apprentice to an engineering firm but *"the early hours and physical labour required compelled him to turn to less exacting work"*. Accordingly, he studied chemistry but then changed to medicine, acquiring the *Licentiate of the Society of Apothecaries* in 1869. This would have allowed him to practise, but he went instead to the University of Aberdeen to graduate in medicine there in 1871. *"He considered going into private practice, but, an opportunity arising, he was appointed assistant demonstrator of anatomy in 1872"*. He continued in this field and in the meantime was elected to the office of assistant surgeon in 1881. Immediately afterwards he was appointed demonstrator of *orthopaedic* surgery, which he held until his appointment as full surgeon in 1897. At this point he exchanged his lectureship in anatomy for one in surgery. He was elected surgeon to the Metropolitan Hospital where he took charge of the department for diseases of the *throat*, but of course is best known to us for his *nasal* surgery and forceps. In addition to these varied feats, his anonymous obituarist considered that *"...he was beautifully made and in perfect proportion"*.[316]

The newcomer to the specialty of otolaryngology, or to give it the full title *otorhinolaryngology* often hears the claims and counter-claims of generalists versus super-specialists and it might be reassuring for him to know that way back in 1910 these problems were exercising the minds of the greatest of the profession such as Watson Williams:

> *But things are very different from what they were when I started practice, and hardly any individual is capable of a complete mastery of the whole range of rhino-laryngology; and if otology be superadded the ground is so extensive that, without devoting his whole time and attention to these subjects over several*

years, no one can hope to be a scientific expert throughout such a large territory.[317]

The same author considered that for an ENT surgeon to master all this equalled, if not surpassed, the requirements for study for the higher examinations in other subjects and awaited the day when an exam and diploma specific to our specialty would be available. Watson Williams' words bear repeating:

> *Surely the practitioner who so qualifies himself for work in laryngo-otology should have the opportunity of being tested by examination and of obtaining his higher degree in this department. He would be better equipped for making the utmost use of his riper clinical experience than by devoting himself, instead, to acquiring an exact knowledge of the anatomy of the whole body and the whole range of advanced medicine or general surgery, at the expense of systematic liberal study of his specialty and all that pertains to it.*

This is all very interesting for us today when audiological medicine is becoming well established and there are moves to transfer emphasis back into the community. The reader might be forgiven if feeling a little confused when he reads that the very same author should have considered that "general practice[nnn] was as good a taking-off ground" as pure surgery. We want contributions from all points of view, and it should always be open to every practitioner to specialize in any direction according to his opportunities for so doing[318]. There does seem some inconsistency in this. Only the most cynical would consider that his views reflected power struggles with the general surgeons and their strangle-hold on the colleges and institutions. Thank goodness nothing like that could ever happen nowadays!

The advice of Watson-Williams of the value of a broadly-based education was found not to be the case even in the 1980s when one of the authors (JDCB) embarked upon the study of paediatrics in order to better his practice of otolaryngology. Success in achieving the Diploma in Child Health was marred a little by the news that refund of expenses etc by his employers would not be forthcoming as this was confined to

---

[nnn] He was quite safe in making this point for Sir James Douglas-Grant (1854-1946) had previously been a G.P. and Dan McKenzie (1874-1936) had spent many years in general practice in Lanarkshire before going to London, where he became editor of the *Journal of Laryngology and Otology*.

professional exams *and by profession he was an otolaryngologist, not a paediatrician!*[319] The embarkation upon a course of study in a related specialty was regarded in similar vein to the Faringdon Folly. This was constructed by Lord Berners, a writer and diplomat who in 1935 built at his home in Oxfordshire, Faringdon House, a 140 foot tower of his own design which had *the great point of being entirely useless.* To discourage anyone who thought of one obvious use for it he put up a notice saying:

> *Members of the public committing suicide from this tower do so at their own risk.*[320]

The problems of education have not gone unnoticed within the corridors of power. The General Medical Council announced in 1991 that it believed that *"increasing specialisation within medicine and the development of postgraduate medical education are among the biggest influences on the way we train doctors".*[321] The challenges facing the profession were eagerly adopted by those whose calling was to write and agitate, rather than treat patients. A representative sentence will suffice to give the flavour of the possible things to come:

> *By removing much of the factual load from the undergraduate medical curriculum we can clear space for topics like communication skills, teamwork, audit, appreciation of scientific method, ethics, information technology etc.*[322]

The views of the authors (including one mother) are too well known to the reader to bear repetition here.

It is perhaps at this moment that your authors should lighten the tone of what might to some of our younger readers (by which we, of course, mean men in their thirties, and for the very unlucky, forties) who are still having to sit examinations might be becoming overwhelmingly melancholic. Certainly the junior author, who despite a veritable alphabet of letters after his name, is in this position is hearing the "black dog" barking. Our mood lightener, once again, concerns the redoubtable Esme Hadfield and the story told to us how whilst up (or, as we Yorkshiremen usually say down) in London to act as examiner for the final FRCS examination she decided not to return to her hotel to spend a boring evening marking scripts. Instead she went straight to Lords to indulge her love of cricket, taking the papers wrapped up in the sealed khaki canvas bag. Even better, she realised that by sitting on the bag she could dispense with the cushion which can be hired, thus saving the expense. Unfortunately on return by taxi to her hotel she found she was in possession of, not a package of examination scripts, but a seat cushion. Throwing this in disgust through the open window, she ordered the driver to return to the cricket ground where, fortunately, the khaki canvas bag was where it had been left, on the terrace. And a good thing too, for, in her own words:

Had I lost all those exam papers the College would have had me by the balls!

But what use is education and training if one cannot convey the fruits of one's efforts to others? That great scientist Ernest Rutherford (who did much of his work in Manchester) held that

A good scientific theory should be explicable to a barmaid.

It was at this point that your authors were going to have a photograph of them attempting to convey some of their scientific intentions to a couple of barmaids - but it never came to pass.

(c) Publish and be Praised.

It will not have gone unnoticed amongst our readers that there has been an ever-increasing pressure upon doctors to publish their research, other people's research, interesting cases - in fact to get their name into print in any way imaginable in order to achieve professional advancement. It is a sort of reverse censorship. In fact it is nothing new - Sigmund Freud was under a similar pressure (which may explain a lot) but of late it seems to have become much worse. The value of publishing articles was impressed upon Freud when he visited Doctor Nothnagel. He asked him whether on the strength of his existing publications he should apply for the *Dozentur*, or whether he should have more. The good doctor merely glanced at the number before pronouncing:

You seem to have eight or nine - oh by all means send in your application.[323]

It is as if the very fact that one has written something down and then persuaded someone else to publish it is proof enough of surgical dexterity, clinical acumen, or whatever is required to be a successful otolaryngologist. Yet journalists, who spend most of their non-drinking hours in this very activity are not universally thought of as especially wise or deserving. Witness the conversation overheard between two of them recently when the first remarked that he would make a mental note of the point. The second coldly remarked: "On what?". It is not as if the bulk of the published material is of any great scientific, or even entertainment value. This was charmingly brought out recently in the *British Medical Journal* where the correspondent recounted how she was advised by a fellow research registrar:

> *Find something to measure, and then keep on measuring it until you can put six points on a graph. Then start submitting extracts, because you will soon be applying for senior registrar jobs and you'll need at least ten publications to get on the short list.*[324]

It does not necessarily follow that getting something published will guarantee success - as many of us are aware. Similarly, a rejection does not always predict unremitting doom. In 1937, *Nature* rejected a submission from Hans Krebs in which he described the linked sequence of enzyme reactions which comprise the citric acid cycle. Instead, it was accepted by a lesser-known journal, *Enzymologia*, and appeared two months later.[325] Krebs was subsequently awarded the Nobel prize and the cycle goes by his name; history does not relate what happened to the editor of *Nature*.

With the increasing number of scientists participating in modern scientific research there is always a problem of attribution of credit. The main author may sometimes conveniently forget the contributions of others who helped. This so-called "quasi-plagiarism" has been the subject of consideration by the International Committee of Medical Ethics (representing 12 medical journals).[326] The manuscripts submitted for publication must now be accompanied by a letter which includes a statement that all the authors approve the paper, as well as providing information on prior or duplicate publications or submissions. One loophole to this, which one of your authors fell through, is when an author submits the work entirely without the knowledge of his fellow workers. He simply signs the form and both the editor and his coworkers are none the wiser until it appears in print under his name alone.[327] It would seem that one should be very cautious. Both your authors were taught to be cautious, and it appears that this teaching extends even to the matter of royal births. Until 1936 and the birth of Princess Alexandra, the

Home Secretary (and members of the Privy Council) were in attendance at the confinement of the Queen or wife of a Prince of the Blood.[328] It must have cost the King (or Civil List) a fair bit for the cigars just to make sure that the Royal Line was kept Royal.

Duplicate publication was condemned in 1984 by Stephen Lock whilst editor of the *British Medical Journal*.[329] In an interview in the *New York Times* (14 December 1982) Benjamin Levin, the editor of *Cell* distinguished three kinds of duplication of articles. There is the situation which arises when under pressure for grants, promotion or tenure the hapless researcher submits simultaneously to several journals the same article for publication. One might call this the shotgun principle. Then, when the time comes and two accept it, it becomes too easy to allow publication in both, thus adding two lines rather than one to the growing curriculum vitae. The second case involves publishing a preliminary report followed later by a more detailed paper which does not materially add to the information contained in the first. Thirdly there is the re-hashing of results already published in primary journals in a collection of papers at a symposium. *The New England Journal of Medicine* led the way in an attempt to stop this practice by introducing in 1969[PPP] the Ingelfinger Rule, named after one of the editors, Franz Ingelfinger. This rule stated in essence that papers were submitted with the understanding that they had been neither published nor submitted elsewhere.[330]

Perhaps it would be instructive to look into some of the emotional roots of such cheating. Chance plays an important role in the choice of a career and should be regarded with just as much weight as the lure of wealth, power or influence or the desire to follow in the family footsteps, important those these may be. Psychological and psychiatric background in the selection of a profession has been discussed by Kubie,[331] a psychiatrist with a wide experience of scientists. He proposes that there are neurotic forces which affect the choice and pursuit of a scientific research career. Your authors would not like to delve too deeply into these psychological/psychiatric rumblings, but, as those of you who have taken the trouble to read so far will be well aware, success and acclaim often

---

PPP

Of course it will come as no surprise to readers of this book that in late 19th century Germany, the problem had already been tackled; research into this area is well underway with one of your authors making trips to Hannover as frequently as his health allows. Look out for the next edition!

bear a relationship to integrity and effort which might be most tactfully described as only "nodding". Those bent on a scientific career are rarely warned that creative capacity, willingness to work hard and even the readiness to make sacrifices in terms of family life and financial reward are not per se sufficient for achievement of success and recognition. One of the authors received advice of quite a different nature from his mother, who, on meeting him on his return from school (he was a Junior Mixed Infant at the time) remonstrated:

> *John, you are weedy. You will have to work very very hard so that you will pass all your exams and be able to get a nice indoor job with no lifting.*

Kubie considers that unresolved anxieties may compel an over anxious investigator to chose a problem that will take a lifetime. However, although negative experiments and the painstaking accumulation of details are important for the advancement of science, they are not the material on which a career can usually be built. It is often a matter of chance whether one remains unknown because of negative results or wins acclaim because of positive ones. At this point one must consider the possibility of giving "chance" a helping hand. Or, in more technical psychological language we can consider that owing to unresolved conflicts and a life lived with a continued "delayed reward" ethos, when a researcher encounters a series of setbacks which delay his progress, he may be tempted to cut corners. For accurate scientific research one needs integrity and honesty. Once you can fake those, you have got it made.

It does perhaps help to have that type of self confidence which will enable one not only to shake off adversity but advertise to the rest of the world one's true worth. Harvey Cushing kept detailed diaries from a very early age, convinced that they would be of benefit to those in the future wanting to write his biography. Of course, Ann Franck did the same, and they make more interesting reading.

REFERENCES

1. Dibble J H. *Napoleon's Surgeon*. London: Heinemann, 1970.
2. Gradenigo G. *Sulla Leptomeningite arcoscritta e sulla paralisi dell'abducente diogigine otica.* Gior. Accad. Med. Torino 1904;10:59.
3. Shambaugh G E. *Surgery of the Ear* Philadephia: W B Saunders, 1967.
4. *Lancet* 1960;ii:656.
5. Weir N *History of Otology.* Br J Audiol 1974;8;113-118.
6. J Laryngol Otol 1951;65:125-126.
7. Mackinlay M S. *Manuel Garcia And His Friends. The Strand Magazine.* 1905;29:257-267.
8. Editorial. *To Señor Manuel Garcia. Punch* 1905;108:208.
9. Wilson J B. *A surgeon's private practice in the nineteenth century.* Medical History 1987;31:349-353.
10. *Obituary Sir William Fergusson. Lancet* 1877;1:258.
11. Semon F. *An Address on the Relations of Laryngology, Rhinology and Otology with other Arts and Sciences.* Br Med J 1904;ii:713-719.
12. Editorial. College of Pathologists. Br Med J 1962;i:1258-1259.
13. *Obituary Sir William Dalby. Lancet* 1919;i:83.
14. *Obituary: Sir Henry Trentham Butlin.* Br Med J 1912;i:276-280.
15. Announcements. Br Med J 1870;i:610.
16. Stevenson R S. *Sir Felix Semon - His Contribution To Laryngology.* Br Med J 1949;ii:1347-1350.
17. *Obituary Sir Felix Semon.* J Laryngol Otol 1921;36:161-162.
18. Editorial. Laryngology at the International Medical Congress. Br Med J 1905;i:673.
19. Shaw H J. *The Life And Times Of The Institute Of Laryngology And Otology.* J Laryngol Otol 1987;101:15-21.
20. Watson Williams P. *Presidential Address.* Proc Roy Soc Med 1910-11;4:1-5.
21. Charnley J. *Super-specialization in Surgery?* Br Med J 1970;2:721-723.
22. Fenton F. *The Ultimate Failure.* Br Med J 1992;305:1027.
23. J Laryngol Otol 1949;63:176-177.
24. Br Med J 1980;2:1149.
25. Editorial. J Med Genetics 1993;30:406-409.
26. Watson Williams P. *Presidential Address.* Proc Roy Soc Med 1910-11;4:1-5.
27. Annotations. *Cardiology as a specialty. Lancet* 1958;ii:1053.
28. Tanner W E. *Sir W Arbuthnot Lane, Bart.* Guy's Hospital Reports 1945;94:85-114.

29. Granshaw L. *Fame and fortune by means of bricks and mortar: the medical profession and specialist hospitals in Britain, 1800-1948.* In: Granshaw L, Porter R (eds) *The Hospital In History.* London: Routledge, 1989.

30. Editorial: *Hospital Distress.* Br Med J 1860;i:458.

31. Clarke J F. *Autobiographical Recollections of the Medical Profession.* London: Churchill, 1874.

32. Editorial: *The Westminster Medical Society and the resignation of the medical officers of the Aldergate Street Dispensary. Lancet* 1833-4;i:218.

33. *Dictionary of National Biography* 1909;17:815-816.

34. Weir N. *History of Otology.* Br J Audiol 1974;8:113-118.

35. Farre J R. *A Treatise on Some Practical Points relating to the Diseases of the Ear by the late John Cunningham Saunders.* London: Longman, Hurst, Rees, Orme & Brown, 1816 (published posthumously).

36. O'Malley J F. *The Tonsillectome - A New Type of Guillotine or Tonsillotome specially designed for the Enucleation of Tonsils.* Proc Roy Soc Med 1912-13;6:51-53.

37. Br Med J 1979;1:1094.

38. J Laryngol Otol 1902;17:629-631.

39. Br Med J 1976;1:776.

40. *Obituary R S Stevenson.* Br Med J 1967;2:58.

41. Young J R. *Radiation Dewlap.* Clin Otol 1979;4:25-28.

42. Finzi N S, Harmer D. *Radium treatment of intrinsic carcinoma of the larynx.* Br Med J 1928;2:886-889.

43. Taylor O. *Florence Cavanagh (obituary)* Br Med J 1992;304:911.

44. Editorial. *Female Medical Students In The United States.* Br Med J 1893;i:47.

45. Medical News. Br Med J 1902;i:1586.

46. Davis N S. *The Higher Education Of Women.* JAMA 1886;7:267-269.

47. Bennett J D C. *The Larger-than-life Story of Princess Doctor Vera Gedroits, Military Surgeon, Poet and Author.* Br Med J 1992;

48. Horne J. *St Blaise.* Proc Roy Soc Med 1927;21:1021.

49. Levin S. *The Speech Defect Of Moses.* J Roy Soc Med 1992;85:632.

50. Cameron H C. *Mr Guy's Hospital.* London: Longman, 1954 p133.

51. *Obituary Hodgkin, Babington. Lancet* 1866;i:445.

52. *Obituary: Dr Babington.* Br Med J 1886;1:447.

53. Rehn L. *Über Penetriende Herzwunden und Herznaht.* Arch Klin Chir 1897;55:315-332.

54. Director Army Surgery AMS Memorandum 52 para 38. DGAMS/19/14/32 of 27 Feb 1990.

55. Ellis H. *Mitchener Memorial Lecture 1988:* July 1 1916. J R Army Med Corps 1989;135:10-12.

56. Bean W B. *Walter Reed and the ordeal of human experiments.* Bull Hist Med 1977;51:75-92.

57. Sternberg M L. *George Miller Sternberg: A Biography.* Chicago: American Medical Association, 1920 p227.

58. Kototkoff N S. K *voprosu metodakh uzstedovaniya Krovanovo devleniya.* Voen med Akad Izvestiia 1905;11:365.

59. Wakerlin G E. *From Bright Toward Light. Circulation* 1962;26:1-6.

60. Freud S. *An Autobiographical Study.* Trans Strachey J. London: Hogarth Press, 1935.

61. Liljestrand G. *Carl Koller and the development of local anaesthesia.* Acta Physiologica Scandinavia 1967 (supplement 299) p25.

62. Watson-Williams P. *New Electric Light Gag for use in Operating on the Facial Regions &c.* Proc Roy Soc Med 1911-12;5:123.

63. Weir N, Weir S, Stephens D. *Who Was Who And What Did They Do?* J Laryngol Otol 1987;101:23-87.

64. *Obituary. Barnsley R E.* J R Army Med Corps 1968;118:78.

65. Self W. *Mentors and Tormentors. The Oldie* 1993;32:25.

66. Bennett J D C, Riddington Young J. *Draffin And His Rods.* J Laryngol Otol 1992;106:1035-1036 (also published, with permission, as *Why Anaesthetists Should Remember Draffin. Today's Anaesthetist* 1993;8:79-80.

67. *Obituary Terence Cawthorne. Lancet* 1970;1:254.

68. McFadzean W A, Bennett J D C. *The Surgeon's Scissor-Jaw Reflex.* Br Med J 1990;301:1428-1429.

69. Bennett J D C. *The Day The Balloon Went Up. Today's Anaesthetist* 1993;8:137.

70. McFadzean W A, Bennett J D C. *The Surgeon's Scissor-Jaw Reflex.* Br Med J 1990;301:1428-1429 (also published, with permission, as Le Réflexe Ciseaux-Mâchoire Du Chirurgien. J.Internat de Médecine 1991;191:47-48).

71. Killian G. *Short hints for examining the oesophagus, trachea, and bronchi by direct methods.* J Laryngol Rhinol Otol 1902;17:505-509.

72. Editorial. *The New Counterblast To Tobacco.* Br Med J 1857;1:133-135.

73. Editorial. *Tobacco Therapy.* Br Med J 1939;1:968.

74. Bennett J D C. *Venereal Disease - The Military Contribution.* Bull Mil Hist Soc 1991;41:123-129.

75. Clifford P. *The Role Of Cytotoxic Drugs.* J Laryngol Otol 1979;93:1151-1180.

76. Botella E. *Sobre los efectos del Salvarsan en el oido interno.* Semana Medica 1913;20:301-304.

77. George G. *On the treatment of epistaxis by the internal administration of ergot.* Br Med J 1876;i:11.

78. Cochrane J. *Treatment of epistaxis.* Br Med J 1876;i:72.

79. Shaer M, Rizk M, Shawaf I, Ali M, Hashash M. *Local Acriflavine: A New Therapy For Rhinoscleroma.* J Laryngol Otol 1981;95:701-706.

80. Price J A. *Hoblyns Dictionary of Medical Terms* London: Whittaker 11th ed, 1887.

81. Bennett J D C, McFarlane H. *Unexpected Factors In "Self-Limiting Ailments"* Br J Clinical Practice 1992;46:210-211.

82. Bennett J D C. Haynes P A. *Non-Medical Prescribing.* J R Army Med Corps 1993;139:73-74.

83. Mythology and Legend. *Funk and Wagnalls Dictionary of European Folklore.* Philadelphia: Funk and Wagnalls, 1949. p334.

84. Valvori A M. *Aspiration of earwigs from metered dose inhaler.* Br Med J 1993;306:797.

85. Taylor J D. *The earwig: the truth about the myth.* Rocky Mt Med J 1978;75:37-38.

86. Fisher J R. *Earwig in the ear.* JAMA 1986;145:245.

87. Hutchins R. Cockroach. In *Encyclopedia Americana.* New York: American Corporation 1971, p167.

88. O'Toole K et al. *Removing Cockroaches from the Auditory Canal: Controlled Trial.* N Engl J Med 1985;312:1197.

89. Warren J et al. *Removing Cockroaches from the Auditory Canal: A Direct Method* N Engl J Med 1989;320:322.

90. Jaffe B F. *The incidence of ear disease in Navaho Indians.* Larygoscope 1969;79:2126.

91. Elias O A. *Lysol Made In England (Letter).* Lancet 1914;ii:668.

92. Bordley J E, Brookhouser P E. *The History of Otology;* in Bradford L J, Hardy W G (eds) *Hearing and Hearing Impairment.* New York: Grune & Stratton, 1979 p6.

93. Politzer A. *Geschichte der Ohrenheilkunde.* Stutgart: Enke Verlag, 1907. Vol 1.

94. McNaughton-Jones H. *Subjective Noises In The Head And Ears: Their Aetiology, Diagnosis And Treatment.* London: Bailliere, Tindall & Cox, 1891.

95. Brown R D, Penny J E, Henley C M, Hodges K B, Kupetz S A, Glenn D W, Jobe P C. *Ototoxic drugs and noise.* In Evered D, Lawrensen G (eds) *Tinnitus Ciba Foundation Symposium 85.* London: Pitman, 1981 p151-171.

96. Lieven W A. *Demonstration of Instruments for the Intravenous Injection of Salvarsan* ("606"). Proc R Soc Med 1910-11;4:45-46.

97. Halstead W S. *Ligature & Suture Material.* JAMA 1913;60:1119-1126.

98. Personal communication to Curt Proskauer *"evidently through the years this material was lost or disposed of".*

99. Watson T. *Lectures on the principles and practice of physic;* delivered at King's College, London. London: John W Parker, 1845 vol 2 p349.

100. Editorial. *Tobacco Therapy.* Br Med J 1939;i:968.

101. Littre E. *Hippocrates: Oevres completes.* Paris: Ballière, 1861.

102. Ross W D. *Works of Aristotle. Historia Animalium.* Oxford: Clarendon, 1910.

103. Peck A L. *Aristotle. Generationis Animalium.* Cambridge: Loeb, 1953.

104. Lederer F L. *The development of otorhinolaryngology and bronchoesophagology.* J Int Coll Surg 1960;33:83-97.

105. *The Papyrus Ebers.* Trans from German by Bryan C P. New York: Appleton, 1971.

106. Bordley J E, Brookhouser P E. *The History of Otology.* In: Bradford L J, Hardy W G (eds) *Hearing and Hearing Impairment.* New York: Grune & Stratton, 1979 p3.

107. O'Malley M H. Bartolomeo Eustachi. *An epistle on the organs of hearing.* Clio Med 1971;6:49-62.

108. Fallopius G. *Observationes Anatomicae.* Venice, 1561.

109. Duverney J G. *Traite de l'organe de l'ouie.* Paris: Michallet, 1683.

110. Asherson N. *Traité de l'Organe de l'Ouie.* J Laryngol Otol 1979;suppl 2.

111. Valsalva A M. *Opera, Hoc Est, Tractatus de Aure Humana.* Venice: Pitteri, 1741.

112. Flourens M. *Experiences sur les canaux semi-circulaires de l'oreille dans les mammiferes.* Memoires de l'Academie des Sciences 1928;9:Oct 13.

113. Menière M P. *Maladies de l'oreille interne offrant les symptomes de la congestion cerebrale apoplectiforme.* Gaz Med Paris 1861;16:597.

114. Menière E. *Quelques considerations sur la maladie du Menière.* 1881. In Wood M. J Laryngol Otol 1968;82:231.

115. Corti A. *Recherches sur l'organe de l'ouie des mammiferes.* Zwiss Zool 1851;3:109-169.

116. Helmholtz H L F. *Die Lehre von den Tenepfindungen als physiologische* Grundlage für die Theorie der Musik. 1863.

117. Mawson S R. *Diseases of the Ear.* London: Butterworth, 1976 3rd ed p166.

118. Bennett J D C. *Downgraded Through My Hearing? Doctor. British Army Review* 1993;105:32-35.

119. Barr T. *Enquiry into the effects of looud sounds upon the hearing of boilermakers and others who work amid noisy suroundings.* Proc Philosophical Soc Glasgow 1886;17:223-239.

120. Bunch C C. *Nerve Deafness Of Known Pathology Or Etiology; Diagnosis Of Occupational Or Traumatic Deafness; Historical And Audiometric Study.* Laryngoscope 1937;47:615-91.

121. Fox S M. *Industrial Noise Exposure and Hearing·Loss.* In Ballenger J J (ed).*Diseases Of The Nose, Throat And Ear.* Philadelphia: Lea & Febiger, 1977 12th ed.

122. Borrett G G. *Protection of Hearing.* J Roy Nav M Serv 1917;3:361.

123. Jobson Horne W. *Gun Deafness And Its Prevention. Lancet* 1914;ii: (Aug 15)

124. Milner S M, Chambers D, Bennett J D C, Stone J. *Antichemical Warfare Tent For Operations In The Gulf.* Br Med J 1991;302:68

125. Milner S M, Chambers D, Bennett J D C. *Surgery In Collective Protection Against Chemical Warfare.* J Roy Coll Surg Edinb 1992;37:118-119.

126. Marriage D. *Warfare Injuries And Neuroses.* Proc Roy Soc Med:53-56.

127. Birkett D. *Warfare Injuries And Neuroses.* Proc Roy Soc Med 1916-17;X (Part iii) Section of Otology:90.

128. Br Med J 1915;i:25 and Br Med J 1915;i:160.

129. Abercrombie P. *Ear Defenders.* Br Med J 1915;i:990.

130. Marriage D. *Warfare Injuries And Neuroses.* Proc Roy Soc Med:53-56.

131. Jobson T B. *Normal Gun-Deafness. Lancet* 1917;ii:566.

132. ISO 4869, SFS 4431,4432, DIN, BSI.

133. Editorial. Br Med J 1972;i:191.

134. Br Med J 1952;ii:233-235.

135. Bennett J D C, Kersebaum M. Noise, *Deafness and the Army. Audiology in Europe* Reading: British Society of Audiology, 1992 p57.

136. Br Med J 1976;i:841.

137. Sydenham R. Air Vice Marshall E D D Dickson. *Hearing* 1979;34:114-116.

138. Reid G. *Further observation on temporary deafness following exposure to gunfire.* J Laryngol Otol 1946:609-633.

139. Fraser J S, Fraser J. *The Morbid Anatomy Of War Injuries Of The Ear.* Proc Roy Soc Med:56-89.

140. Faulks (Mr Justice). Chester Crown Court. Bolton v Hawker Sidderley March 1973.

141. Head P. Minutes, *Triservice Otolaryngological Panel*. Meeting held at the Central Medical Establishment RAF London 4 June 1973 p1 para1.

142. Stevenson R S, Guthrie D. *A History of Otolaryngology*. Edinburgh: Livingstone, 1949.

143. Flint R W. *History of Education for the Hearing Impaired*. Bradford L J and Hardy W G (eds) *Hearing and Hearing Impairment*. New York: Grune and Stratton, 1979.

144. Flint R W. *History of Education for the Hearing Impaired*. In Bradford R L, Hardy W G (eds) *Hearing and Hearing Impairment*. New York: Grune and Stratton, 1979.

145. Garrison F H. *An Introduction To The History Of Medicine*. Philadephia: Saunders, 1929 4th ed.

146. Taylor I G. *Alexander Ewing (1896-1980) Teacher of the Deaf*. p137.

147. Siegel R E. *Galen on Sense Perception*. Basel: Karger, 1970.

148. Stephens S D G. *Personality Tests In Meniere's Disorder*. J Laryngol Otol 1975;89:479-490.

149. King-Hele D. *Erasmus Darwin 1771-1802*. London: Macmillan, 1963. King-Hele D. *Doctor of Revolution*. London: Faber & Faber, 1977.

150. Bárány R. *Untersuchungen über den vom Vestibularapparat des Ohres Reflektorisch Ausgelsten Rhythmishcen Nystagmus und seine Begleiterscheinungen* (Eine Betrag zur Physiologie und Pathologie des Bogengangapparate). Berlin: C Coblenz, 1906.

151. Jenkins G J. Otosclerosis: *Certain clinical features and experimental operative procedures*. Trans XVllth Int Congress Med,(1913) London.

152. Portmann G. *Recherches sur le Sac Endolymphatique: Resultats et Applications Chirurgicales*. Groningen: Collegium Oto-Rhino-Laryngologicum 1926.

153. Dandy W. *Effects on hearing after sub-total section of the cochlear branch of the auditory nerve*. Bull Johns Hopkins Hosp 1934;55:240-243.

154. Dandy W E. *The surgical treatment of Meniere's disease*. Surg Gynecol Obstet 1941;72:421-425.

155. Schuknecht H F. *Ablation therapy in Meniere's disease*. Laryngoscope 1956;66:859-870.

156. Cawthorne T. *Membranous labyrinthectomy via the oval window for Meniere's disease*. J Laryngol Otol 1957;71:524.

157. Arslan M. *Direkt Applikation des Ultrashalls auf das knockerne Labyrinth zur Therapieder Labyrinthose (Morbus Meniere)*. Hals Nasen Ohrenheilk 1954;4:166.

158. Hallpike C S, Cairns H. J Laryngol Otol 1938;53:625.

159. Weir N. *History of Otolaryngology*. British Journal of Audiology. 1974;8:113-118.

160. Forrest D W. *Francis Galton - The Life and Work of a Victorian Genius.* London: Elek, 1974.

161. Stevenson R S, Guthrie D. *A History of Otolaryngology.* Edinburgh: Churchill Livingstone, 1949 p61.

162. Johnson E W. *Tuning Forks To Audiometers And Back Again.* Laryngoscope 1970;80:49-68.

163. Rinne A. *Beitrage zur Physiologie des menschlichen Ohres.* (Contributions to the Physiology of the Human Ear). Vierteljahrschr. prakt. Heilk. Med. Fak. Prag 1855;12:71-123.

164. J Laryngol Otol 1922;37:540-541.

165. Duncanson J J K. *The Electric Telephone as a means of Measuring the Hearing Power.* Br Med J 1878;i:335.

166. *Discussion on Value and Significance of Hearing Tests.* Proc Roy Soc Med 1912;v(Section Otology):113-131.

167. Scott S. *Warfare Injuries and Neuroses.* Proc Roy Soc Med 112.

168. Taylor I G. *Alexander Ewing (1896-1980) Teacher of the Deaf* p137.

169. Wever E G, Lawrence M. *Physiological Acoustics.* Princeton, New Jersey: Princeton University Press, 1954.

170. Békésy G von. *Über die Messung der Schwingungsamplitude der Gehorknochelchen mittels einer kapazititiven Sonde.* Akust Z 1941;6:1-16.

171. Metz D. *The acoustic impedance measured on normal and pathological ears.* Acta Otolaryngol Suppl 1946;63:1-254.

172. Békésy G von. *A new audiometer.* Acta Otolaryngol 1947;35:411-422.

173. Carhart R. *Clinical determination of abnormal auditory adaptation.* Arch Otolaryngol 1957;65:32-39.

174. Clarke J F. *Autobiographical Recollections of the Medical Profession.* London: Churchill, 1874.

175. Young J R. *Aids to Hearing.* Rostrum 1982;105:6-7.

176. Personal communication: Gillian Lacey, at *Audiology in Europe,* the so-called "First European Conference On Audiology".

177. Bordley J E, Brookhouser P E. *The History of Otology.* in Bradford L J, Hardy W G (eds) *Hearing and Hearing Impairment.* New York: Grune & Stratton, 1979 p4.

178. Mettler F A. *History of Medicine.* Philadelphia: Blakiston, 1947.

179. Werner H. *History of the problem of Deaf-Mutism until the 17th century.* Trans orig German text by Bonning C K. 1932.

180. Cleland A. *Instruments proposed to remedy some kinds of deafness.* Philosophical Transactions of the Royal Society 1741;41:848-851.

181. Guyot E G. *Instrument pur seringuer la trompe d'Eustache par la bouche.* Hist Acad Roy Sci 1726.

182. Cleland A. *Instruments to remedy some kinds of deafness.* Phil Trans Roy Soc 1744;41:848.

183. Stevenson R S, Guthrie D. *A History of Otolaryngology.* Edinburgh: Churchill Livingstone, 1949 p61.

184. Allen P. *Lectures on Aural Catarrh and Curable Deafness.* London: Churchill, 1871.

185. Weir N. *History of Otology.* Br J Audiol 1974;8:113-118.

186. Shrapnell H J. London Med Gaz 1832;10:120

187. Cooper A P. Phil Trans Roy Soc 1801;91:435.

188. Weir N. History of Otolaryngology. Br J Audiol 1974;8:113-118.

189. Saunders J C. *The Anatomy of the Human Ear, with a Treatise on the Diseases of that Organ.* London, 1806.

190. Valsalva A M. *De aure humana tractatus.* Bologna 1704.

191. Kessell J. *Über das Mobilisieren des Steigbugels durch Ausschneiden des Tromellfells, Hammers und Ambosses bei Undurchgangigkeit der Tube.* Arch Ohr Nas Kehlkopfheilk 1878;13:69.

192. J Laryngol Rhinol Otol 1904;19:287-288.

193. Ballance C A, Duel A B. Archives of Otolaryngology 1932;15:70.

194. Holmgren G. *Some experiences in surgery for otosclerosis.* Acta Otolaryngol 1923;5:460-466.

195. Sourdille M. *New technique on the surgical treatment of severe and progressive deafness from otosclerosis.* Bull N Y Acad Med 1937;13:673-691.

196. Holmgren G. *The surgery of otosclerosis.* Ann Oto Rhinol Laryngol 1937;46:6-12.

197. Lempert J. *Improvement of hearing in cases of otosclerosis: new, one-stage surgical technic.* Arch Otolaryngol 1938;65:302-331.

198. Anonymous obituary. *The Daily Telegraph* 23 October 1991 p21.

199. Obituary. *Lancet* 1970;i:254.

200. Rosen S. *Mobilisation of the stapes to restore hearing in otosclerosis.* NY J Med 1953;53:2650-2653.

201. Shea J J. *Fenestration of the oval window.* Ann Otol Rhinol Laryngol 1958;67:932-951.

202. Rosen S. *None So Deaf.* London: W H Allen, 1973 p171.

203. Brock A J (transl.) *The Works of Galen.* London: Loeb Classical Library, 1916.

204. Riolanus J. *Opera anatomica.* Paris, 1649.

205. Petit J L. *Traite des maladies chirurgicales.* Paris, 1774.

206. Simpson J F. *Joseph Toynbee - his contributions to otology.* Proc R Soc Med 1963;56:97-105.

207. McFarland G E. *A Brief History fo Otolaryngology.* Trans Am Acad Ophthal Otolaryngol 1974;78:115-120.

208. Willemot J et al. Histoire de L'ORL. Acta Oto-Rhino-Laryngologica Belgica 1981:602.

209. Stevenson R S, Guthrie D. *A History of Otolaryngology.* Edinburgh: Churchill Livingstone, 1949 p61.

210. Tanner W E. *Sir Arbuthnot Lane, Bart.* Guy's Hospital Reports 1945;94:85-114.

211. *Lancet* 1893;i:991.

212. *Lancet* 1891;i:83.

213. Hammond V. *Disease of the external ear.* In Kerr A G (ed) *Scott Brown's Otolaryngology.* London: Butterworths, 1987 vol 3 p170.

214. Van Gilse P H G. *Des observations ulterieures sur la genese des exostoses due conduit externe par l'irritation d'eau froids.* Acta Otolaryngologica 1938;26:343-352.

215. Fowler E P Jnr, Osman P M. *New Bone Growth Due To Cold Water In Ears.* Arch Otolaryngol 1942;36:455-466.

216. Harrison D F N. *The relationship of osteomata of the external auditory meatus to swimming.* Annals Roy Coll Surg Eng 1962;31:187-202.

217. Timpson J. *English Eccentrics.* Norwich: Jarrold, 1991. p150-151

218. Editorial. Br Med J 1902;i:161.

219. Robson AK, Leighton SEJ, Anslow P, Milford CA. *MRI as a single procedure for acoustic neuroma: a cost effective protocol.* J Roy Soc Med 1993;86:455-457.

220. Stack JP, Ramsden RT, Antoun NM, Lye RH, Isherwood I, Jenkins JPR. *Magnetic Resonance Imaging of acoustic neuromas; the role of gadolinium-DPTA.* Br J Radiol 1988;61:800-805.

221. Sandifort, Edward. *Observationes Anatomico Pathological.* Lugduni Batavorum. 1771. ch IX pp 116-121

222. McMinn (ed) *Last's Textbook of Anatomy.* The biographical notes were compiled by Jessie Dobson, a curator at the Royal College of Surgeons.

223. Schrapnell. *Das Bertelsmann Lexikon.* Gutersloh: Das Bertelsmann Verlag 1974 vol 9 p 24.

224. Shrapnell-Membran. *Pschyrembel Klinisches Wörterbuch*. Berlin: Walter de Gruyter, 1990 p1539.

225. *Obituary.* Br Med J 1969;297:551-552

226. *Obituary.* Br Med J 1945;i:279.

227. J Laryngol Otol 1946;61:41.

228. Dundas Grant J. *Warfare Injuries And Neuroses*. Proc Roy Soc Med 1916-17;X (Part iii) Section of Otology: 93-96.

229. Rolls R. *Archibald Cleland: c1700-1771*. Br Med J 1984;288:1132-1134.

230. Timpson J. *English Eccentrics*. Norwich: Jarrold, 1991 p150-151.

231. Derbes V J. *The Keepers of the Bed*. JAMA 1970;212:97-100.

232. Clarkson P. *Sir Harold Gillies*. Br Med J 1966;ii:641.

233. Bennett J D C. *Medical Advances Consequent To The Great War 1914-1918*. J Roy Soc Med 1990;83:738-742.

234. Till A S. *Gordon-Taylor, war surgeon and historian*. Ann R Coll Surg 1974;54:33-47.

235. Wallace A F. *The Development Of Plastic Surgery For War*. J R Army Med Corps 1985;131:28-37.

236. J Laryngol Otol 1938;53:812.

237. Br Med J 1971;i:574.

238. Bennett J D C. *Medical Support For British 8th Army World War Two. Army History* (in print).

239. Sydenham R. Air Vice Marshall E D D Dickson. *Hearing* 1979;34:114-116.

240. Fraser I. The Mitchiner Memorial Lecture: *The Doctor's Debt To The Soldier*. J Roy Army Med Corps 1972;118:1-16.

241. Tagliacozzi G. *De curtorum chirurgia per insitionem*. Venice:1579.

242. Wallace A F. *The Progress of Plastic Surgery*. Oxford: Meeus, 1982.

243. Lucas B. *Gentleman's Magazine* 1794;Oct:891.

244. Almant S C. *Rhinoplasty in Kangra. Nose-making since Moghul period*. Punj Med J 1967;16:287-293.

245. Notes and Queries. *Guardian* 1992;2:10-11 (4 Dec).

246. Adams F (trans). *The Works of Paul Aeginata*. London 3 vols 1846-47.

247. Fallopius G. *Observationes Anatomicae*. Venice, 1561.

248. Babington B G. *Lancet* 1865;ii:362.

249. Sutton H G. *Medical Mirror* 1864;1:769.

250. Cochrane J. *Treatment of Epistaxis*. Br Med J 1876;i:72.

251. Kisch H A. *The Rhinomanometer*. Proc Roy Soc Med 1913-14;7:19.

252. Br Med J 1910;i:1271.

253. *Any Questions?* Br Med J 1952;ii:454.

254. Willemot et al. Histoire de L'ORL. Acta Oto-Rhino-Laryngologica Belgica.

255. Highmore N. *Corporis Humani Disquisito Anatomica*. The Hague 1651.

256. Stevenson R S, Guthrie D. *A History of Otolaryngology*. Edinburgh: Livingstone, 1949.

257. Whymper W. *The gunner with the silver mask: Being an extraordinary case of extensive destruction of the lower jaw by a shell. London Medical Gazette* 1832/ 33;12:705-709.

258. Ballingall Sir George. *Cases & communications illustrative of subjects in military and naval surgery.* Edin Med & Surg J 1842;57:116-121.

259. St Clair Thomson, Negus. *Diseases of the Nose and Throat*. London: Cassell, 1955 p432.

260. Spencer W (transl) *De Medicina* ii, 12. London: Loeb Classical Library, 1935.

261. St Clair Thomson, Negus. *Diseases of the Nose and Throat*. London: Cassell 1955 p363.

262. St Clair Thomson, Negus. *Diseases of the Nose and Throat*. London: Cassell, 1955 p359.

263. Desault P J. *Oevres chirurgicales de Desault* (edited by Bichat). Paris, 1798.

264. Tanner W E. Sir Arbuthnot Lane, Bart. Guy's Hospital Reports 1945;94:85-114.

265. Hoblyn R D. *A Dictionary of Terms used in Medicine*. London: Whittaker, 1887 11th ed.

266. *The Faber Medical Dictionary*. London: Faber & Faber, 1953.

267. Martine G. Phil Trans Roy Soc 1730; p 448.

268. Habermann G. *Stimme u Sprache*. Stuttgart: Georg Thieme Verlag, 1978.

269. Italian Medicine Department. BMA News Review 1993;19(7):33.

270. *Lancet* 1855;i:331.

271. J Laryngol Otol 1953;67:90-97.

272. Gibb G D. *The first attempt in England to remove a growth from the larynx through division of the Pomum Adami.* Br Med J 1865;ii:327-331.

273. Gibb G D. *On diseases of the throat and windpipe* London: Churchill, 1864.

274. Huxham J. *A Dissertation on the Malignant, Ulcerous Sore Throat*. London, 1757.

275. Tanner W E. *Sir Arbuthnot Lane, Bart.* Guy's Hospital Reports 1945;94:85-114.

276. Personal communication Stephen M Milner, who assisted Dr Hendren when they worked together at the Shriners' Burns Institute, Boston U.S.A.

277. Alexander A B. *? Otitic Barotrauma.* Br Med J 1945;1:276.

278. Brown Kelly H D. *What's In A Name.* J Roy Soc Med 1992;85:585.

279. Bennett J D C. *Lesions Of The Internal Auditory Meatus (letter).* J Roy Soc Med 1993;87:245.

280. Martin A H. *Inferior Turbinates (letter).* J Roy Soc Med 1992;85:511.

281. Padgham N, Vaughan-Jones R. *Inferior Turbinates (reply to letter).* J Roy Soc Med 1992;85:511.

282. Warning to Civil Defence Workers - the strict laws of the land preclude our revealing the exact source of this for reasons of National Security.

283. Vinson P P. *Hysterical Dysphagia.* Minn Med 1922;5:107.

284. Paterson D R. Proc Roy Soc Med 1918-1919;12:235.

285. Kelly A Brown. Proc Roy Soc Med 1918-1919;12:235.

286. Bronner A. *Notes on some cases of painful fissure of the mouth of the oesophagus.* J Laryngol Otol 1913;28:32-34.

287. Thomas J. *Doctor Or Mister, What's In A Name.* Hospital Doctor 1992;Jan:40.

288. *A Doctor, But Not M.D.* Br Med J 1876;1:90-91.

289. Medical News. Br Med J 1902;1:1586.

290. Announcements. Br Med J 1870;i:610.

291. Mott F. *Appetite and Digestion.* In Craig E (ed) *Cookery Illustrated and Household Management.* London: Odhams, 1936.

292. O'Malley J F. *The Tonsillectome - A New Type of Guillotine or Tonsillotome specially designed for the Enucleation of Tonsils.* Proc Roy Soc Med 1912-13;6:51-53.

293. Personal communication Kenneth Harrison (who was appalled to hear this from a patient).

294. Bennett A. *A Woman Of No Importance.*

295. Shambaugh G E. *Surgery of the Ear.* Philadelphia: W B Saunders, 1967 2nd ed. p160.

296. Laerum O D, Skullerud K. *Morbidity in assistants at surgical operations.* Can Med Assoc J 1974;110:632-635.

297. Stevenson R S, Guthrie D. *A History of Otolaryngology* Edinburgh: Churchill Livingstone, 1949.

298. Baden-Powell *Rovering To Success.* 1922.

299. O'Malley J F. *The Tonsillectome - A New Type of Guillotine or Tonsillotome specially designed for the Enucleation of Tonsils.* Proc Roy Soc Med 1912-13;6:51-53.

300. Thomson St Clair. *The Treatment Of Adenoids (letter).* Br Med J 1905;i:279.

301. *Obituary Lennox Browne.* J Laryngol Otol 1902;17:629-631.

302. Sherrington C. *Sir Charles Ballance.* Lancet 1936;i:396.

303. *Obituary Mr Arthur H Cheatle.* J Laryngol Otol 1929;44:424-425.

304. Editorial. Edinburgh Medical and Surgical Journal 1814;10:104-116.

305. *Obituary Sir Henry Trentham Butlin.* Br Med J 1912;1:276-280.

306. *Obituary James Taylor* Br Med J 1912;i:281.

307. Butlin H T. *A Clinical Lecture on Oophorectomy In The Treatment of Cancer of the Breast.* Br Med J 1902;i:10-13.

308. McKenzie D. *Tubes of Soft Metal for Insertion into Nose after Submucous Resection.* Proc Roy Soc Med 1914-15;8:49.

309. Bennett J D C, Riddington Young J. *Draffin And His Rods.* J Laryngol Otol 1992;106:1035-36 (also published, with permission, as *Why Anaesthetists Should Remember Draffin. Today's Anaesthetist* 1993;8:79-80.

310. Clarke J F. *Autobiographical Recollections of the Medical Profession.* London: Churchill, 1874.

311. Merrington W R. *University College Hospital and its Medical School: a History.* London: Heinemann, 1976. p158.

312. Announcements. Br Med J 1876;i:265.

313. Joiner C L. *Babington's Syndrome - Setting The Record Straight.* Br J Clin Pract 1992;46:198-202.

314. Independent on Sunday 1993;28 May p3.

315. Mott F. *Appetite and Digestion.* In Craig E (ed) *Cookery Illustrated and Household Management.* London: Odhams, 1936.

316. *Obituary William Johnson Walsham.* Lancet 1903;ii:1122-1125.

317. Watson Williams P. *Presidential Address.* Proc Roy Soc Med 1910-11;4:1-5.

318. Watson Williams P. *Presidential Address.* Proc Roy Soc Med 1910-11;4:1-5.

319. ERB Form No 1. Application For Travel/Subsistence At Public Expense. 7 Aug 1987.

320. Timpson J. *English Eccentrics.* Norwich: Jarrold 1991.

321. General Medical Council. *Undergraduate Medical Education.* London: GMC, 1991. (Discussion document by working party of GMC Education Committee).

322. Lowry S (assistant editor). *Trends in health care and their effects on medical education.* Br Med J 1993;306:255-258.

323. Freud S. *Letter to Martha Bernays 16 Jan 1885. Letters of Sigmund Freud 1873-1938* (ed) Freud E L. London: The Hogarth Press, 1961.

324. Greenhalgh T. *Publish or Perish.* Br Med J 1991;303;1556.

325. Dixon B. *The Grossest Failures Of Peer Review.* Br Med J 1993;307:137.

326. International Committee of Medical Journal Editors. Br Med J 1985;291:722.

327. Bennett J D C. *An Agreement Of Intent.* Br Med J 1991;303:996.

328. The duties of the Home Secretary on the occasion of a Royal birth. Archive 108/50, library of the Royal College of Physicians.

329. Lock S. *Repetitive publication: a waste that must stop.* Br Med J 1984;288:661.

330. Editorial. New Eng J Med 1969;281:676.

331. Kubie L S. *Some unresolved problems of the scientific career.* Am Scientist 1953;10:596 and 1954;1:104.